The Alexandrian Summaries of Galen's *On Critical Days*

Islamic Philosophy, Theology and Science

TEXTS AND STUDIES

Edited by

Hans Daiber
Anna Akasoy
Emilie Savage-Smith

VOLUME 92

The titles published in this series are listed at *brill.com/ipts*

The Alexandrian Summaries of Galen's *On Critical Days*

Editions and Translations of the Two Versions of the Jawāmiʿ*, with an Introduction and Notes*

By

Gerrit Bos
Y. Tzvi Langermann

BRILL

LEIDEN | BOSTON

Cover Illustration: Cod. Parma 2919; De Rossi 1276; Richler 1498. The MS, missing foliation, was copied in the fifteenth century in a Byzantine script; in the right and bottom margin of the beginning of Book two it has the Hebrew term: המבשרים (the indicators [of the crisis]). Reproduced with the permission of Ministry of Cultural Heritage and Activities (Italy).

Library of Congress Cataloging-in-Publication Data

Galen.
[De diebus decretoriis. Arabic. Selections]
The Alexandrian summaries of Galen's On critical days : editions and translations of the two versions of the Jawami' / with an introduction and notes by Gerrit Bos, Y. Tzvi Langermann.
pages cm. -- (Islamic philosophy, theology and science ; v. 92)
Includes bibliographical references and index.
ISBN 978-90-04-28221-6 (hardback : alk. paper) -- ISBN 978-90-04-28222-3 (e-book)
1. Galen. De diebus decretoriis. 2. Prognosis--Early works to 1800. 3. Medicine, Greek and Roman. 4. Medicine, Arab. 5. Medical astrology--Early works to 1800. I. Bos, Gerrit, 1948- II. Langermann, Y. Tzvi. III. Galen. De diebus decretoriis. English. IV. Galen. De diebus decretoriis. Hebrew. V. Title.

R126.G33 2015
610.938--dc23

2014036501

This publication has been typeset in the multilingual "Brill" typeface. With over 5,100 characters covering Latin, IPA, Greek, and Cyrillic, this typeface is especially suitable for use in the humanities. For more information, please see www.brill.com/brill-typeface.

ISSN 0169-8729
ISBN 978-90-04-28221-6 (hardback)
ISBN 978-90-04-28222-3 (e-book)

Printed by Printforce, the Netherlands

Contents

Preface

Galen was undoubtedly the most important medical authority in antiquity, and one of the most influential medical authorities of all times. He bequeathed an enormous body of writings, mostly, but by no means all, in the field of medicine. His works were translated into Syriac, then into Arabic, by the Christian physicians of the early Abbasid period who played a pivotal role in the transmission of the Galenic corpus to the Arabic-speaking world. Galen's works were translated into Latin, either directly from the Greek or by way of the Arabic, and formed the basis of university and extra-university medicine in medieval and Renaissance Europe. Galenic medicine is the basis of the tremendous, wide-ranging, and often innovative writings of medieval Muslim, Christian, and Jewish physicians who wrote in the principal scientific languages of the medieval world—Arabic, Hebrew, Latin, Persian, and Syriac.

However, translations of books authored by the master were not the only vehicle by which "Galenic" medicine exercised its enormous impact. Galen was anything but concise, and he was prone to digressions and polemical excursuses. For that reason, already in late antiquity, some sixteen Galenic treatises were selected for a sort of "core curriculum" for the medical student. But this is not all. There exists a group of "summaries", often referred to as the "Alexandrian summaries" (*Jawāmiʿ al-Iskandarāniyīn*, Summaria Alexandrinorum), which overlap for the most part with the curriculum of sixteen books which were taught with formal commentaries and read in a specific order in pre-Islamic Alexandria and in the early centuries of Islam.[1] Though there has always been a suspicion that the summaries were written originally in Greek, perhaps in Alexandria, no Greek texts are known to exist. The texts we publish here furnish some new information on the literary history of the "summaries", though the question of their origin remains open.

As the name implies, these are greatly abridged versions of the Galenic originals. However, they do not merely shorten the exposition; they maintain a certain critical distance from Galen, introducing as well minor, and at times even major, revisions of Galenic doctrine. As such they are entirely distinct from the *Epitomes* of the core curriculum prepared, for example, by Maimonides, who tells us explicitly that he has built the abridgements by piecing together literal quotations from Galen.[2]

1 The literature on this body of texts is not very extensive, but interest has grown in recent years. See the bibliography.

2 See Maimonides, *Medical Aphorisms, Treatises 1-5*, ed. and trans. Gerrit Bos (Provo, 2004),

Galen's writings were thus transformed, not just by crossing linguistic boundaries, but by deliberate intervention on the part of unnamed medical writers who felt the need to adjust Galen's teachings. There is evidence that at least in some cases, it was the revised Galen transmitted by the summaries, rather than the original Galen, that entered into the medieval discourse.

In the present publication we present editions and translations of the summaries to Galen's *On Critical Days*. Two very different versions exist, the one in Arabic, the other in a Hebrew translation from a lost Arabic text. Moreover, there are some significant differences between the two extant copies of the Arabic text. Some of the key differences between the teachings of the summaries and those of Galen have already been discussed by one of us.[3] We introduce the present study with a thorough conspectus of the two summaries, in particular calling attention to where they diverge from Galen, seeing as our main interest in this study is the transformation of Galen in the summaries; the subsequent impact of the summaries must be left to another project. For purposes of comparison we have used the recent edition and translation of Ḥunayn's translation of *On Critical Days* by Glenn Cooper;[4] page numbers are indicated by (CG pp.). Where warranted, Kühn's edition of the Greek has also been consulted;[5] page and line numbers are indicated by [K ppp:ll]. For convenience of reference the texts have been divided into numbered passages indicated by square brackets [].

We wish to thank the libraries whose resources were made available for this publication: Princeton University Library, Majlis Library in Tehran, Bibliothèque Nationale de France, Biblioteca Palatina in Parma, National Library of Russia, and the Österreichische Nationalbiliothek. Thanks go out as well to the Insitute of Microfilmed Hebrew Manuscripts in Jerusalem and its

---

p. 2: "In these aphorisms I have not followed the method that I followed in the *Epitomes*, in which I quoted Galen's very words, as I stipulated in the introduction to the *Epitomes*." Maimonides' *Epitomes* are extant in a beautiful manuscript at Paris, BNF héb 1203, including some notes added by Maimonides to the *Epitomes*; see Y. Tzvi Langermann, "Maimonides on the Synochous Fever," *Israel Oriental Studies* 12 (1993), 175-198.

3 Y. Tzvi Langermann, "The Astral Connections of Critical Days: Some Late Antique Sources Preserved in Hebrew and Arabic," in Anna Akasoy, Charles Burnett and Ronit Yoeli-Tlalim (eds.), *Astromedicine, Astrology, and Medicine, East and West* (Florence, 2008), 99-118.

4 Cf. C.M. Cooper, *Galen*, De diebus decretoriis, *from Greek into Arabic. A Critical Edition, with Translation and Commentary, of Ḥunayn Ibn Isḥāq*, Kitāb ayyām al-buḥrān (Farnham-Burlington, 2011).

5 Cf. C.G. Kühn, *Claudii Galeni Opera Omnia*, 20 vols. (Leipzig, 1821-1833, repr. Hildesheim, 1967).

staff. Our thanks are extended to Dr. Leigh Chipman for her valuable help in preparing these texts. Research for this project was carried out with the generous support of the German-Israel Foundation (Research Grant I-1053-110.4/2009), which we acknowledge with profound thanks.

CHAPTER 1

The "Summaries" and Other Recensions of Galen

The collection referred to, properly or not, as the Alexandrian summaries of Galen, has attracted interest for several generations.[1] They promise, on account of their purported Alexandrian origins, to be an important source for the transmission of Greek wisdom "from Alexandria to Baghdad". The total absence of any trace of Greek originals for the collection has deepened the mystery surrounding them. In this first section of our introduction we will briefly review the main texts and issues, as well as taking note of some of the most recent research. However, our main purpose here, as, indeed, it is one of the major objectives of the publication of the Arabic and Hebrew texts in this volume, is to establish what these summaries were about; and we include here not just those that are said in their titles to be "Alexandrian summaries", but other epitomes as well. Examples of the latter include the collection ascribed to "Yaḥyā al-Naḥwī" and the recently discovered summary of *On the Elements According to Hippocrates* attributed to Ḥunayn bin Isḥāq.[2] All of these belong to the same genre as the Alexandrian summaries and were written with the same aims in mind.

These writings had two main objectives: (1) Making Galen's books more accessible, especially for students; (2) Bringing Galen up-to-date. There is no surprise or controversy concerning the first of these. Galen is one of the most prolix authors of all times, and his books are full of long diversions, which, for all of their interest, were something that medical students could do without. The second objective is not yet fully appreciated. The summaries—both those said to be Alexandrian and those not—are not just shortened versions of Galen; they display some revision which at times may even be in flagrant contradiction to what Galen had taught.

The most important description of the history of these texts, and their

---

1 Research up to the last decades of the twentieth century and, more importantly, a list of manuscripts, can be found in Fuat Sezgin, *Geschichte des arabischen Schrifttums* (Leiden, 1970), 3: 140-150, 4: 405-408; 7: 376-377; and Manfred Ullmann, *Die Medizin im Islam* (Leiden, 1970), 65-67, 343. Their accounts wisely include the various epitomes and recensions ascribed to Yaḥyā al-Naḥwī, Abū al-Faraj Ibn al-Ṭayyib, and Ibn Zurʿa, and not just those attributed to unnamed "Alexandrians".

2 See the preceding note; on the newly found epitome by Ḥunayn, see Gerrit Bos and Y. Tzvi Langermann, "An Unknown Summary of Galen's *On the Elements According to Hippocrates*, attributed to Ḥunayn Ibn Isḥāq," forthcoming in *Arabic Sciences and Philosophy*.

 | DOI 10.1163/9789004282223_002

reception and study among the Christians of Baghdad, remains that provided by the "Meisterübersetzer", Ḥunayn ibn Isḥāq, himself a Christian of Baghdad. We reproduce it here in the translation of M. Meyerhof:

> These (Nos. 1-20) are the books to the reading of which the students of the Medical School at Alexandria were confined. They used to read them in the order which I have followed in my list. They were accustomed to meet every day for the reading and interpretation of one of the standard works, in the same way in which, in our days, our Christian friends are accustomed to meet every day at the educational institution known as σκολή for the study of a standard work from among the books of the Ancients. Concerning the remainder of (GALEN's) books they were accustomed to read them everyone for himself, after an introductory study of the aforementioned books; just as our friends read today the explanations of the books of the Ancients.[3]

Recent studies by Gregor Schoeler and Gotthard Strohmaier have called into question Meyerhof's reading of this text, according to which the Christian schools as well as the Bayt al-Ḥikma of Baghdad were in some way at least a direct continuation of the Alexandrian schools of late antiquity.[4] This line of inquiry is not of particular interest to the present study; even less though is the deeper critique of Meyerhof's Alexandria to Baghdad narrative.[5] Neither

3 Max Meyerhof, "New light on Ḥunain Ibn Isḥâq and his period," *Isis 8* (1926), 685-724, at p. 702. The Arabic text was published by G. Bergsträsser, *Ḥunain ibn Isḥâq über die syrischen und arabischen Galen-Übersetzungen* (Abhandlungen für die Kunde des Morgenlandes, XVII, 2; Leipzig, 1925). See also F. Käs, *Eine neue Handschrift von Ḥunain ibn Isḥāqs Galenbibliographie* (Zeitschrift für Geschichte der arabisch-islamischen Wissenschaften 19; Frankfurt am Main, 2011).

4 Gregor Schoeler, "Die Frage der schriftlichen oder mündlichen Überlieferung der Wissenschaften im frühen Islam," *Der Islam 62* (1985), 201-230; idem, "Weiteres zur Frage der schriftlichen oder mündlichen Überlieferung der Wissenschaften im Islam," *Der Islam 66* (1989), 38-67; Gotthard Strohmaier, "Die christlichen Schulen in Baghdad und der alexandrinische Kanon der Galenschriften. Eine Korrektur in Ḥunains Sendschreiben an 'Alī ibn Yaḥyā," *Oriens 36* (2001), 268-275. One should also mention the study of Albert Z. Iskandar, "An attempted reconstruction of the late Alexandrian medical curriculum," *Medical history 20* (1976), 235-258, which supplements the materials adduced by Meyerhof with information from other sources. Recent research greatly downplays the role of the Bayt al-Ḥikma; see Dimitri Gutas, *Greek Thought, Arabic Culture: The Graeco-Arabic Translation Movement in Baghdad and Early 'Abbasaid Society (2nd-4th/5th-10th c.)* (London, 2012), 58-59.

5 We refer of course to the classic study of Max Meyerhof, *Von Alexandrien nach Bagdad: Ein Beitrag zur Geschichte des philosophischen und medizinischen Unterrichts bei den Ara-*

the purported Alexandrian origins of the summaries, nor the vexed question of the continuity of school traditions, are pivotal questions for our study. We are rather interested mainly in the scientific and doctrine content of the summaries, and we are on the lookout for modifications of or deviations from Galen's original teachings—revisions that may have helped shape the particular forms "Galenism" would take in Islamicate culture.

Let us then turn to our main subject of interest, the content of the summaries and their differences with the original Galen. Focusing on an important anatomical text, Albert Z. Iskandar notes some differences in organization and content between the summaries and Galen; Ḥunayn takes them to be deliberate changes made by "the Alexandrians".[6] As the title of his paper reveals, Iskandar is interested mainly in bibliography. He observes:

> Ḥunain points to some title-differences in Greek manuscripts of Galen's *De venarum arteria-rumque dissectione* for which, he remarks, the Alexandrians are responsible. Further, he throws light on the origin of his own Arabic translation which seems to have descended from versions used by the Alexandrians. While the Greek text is in one treatise, Arabic manuscripts exist invariably in two treatises: *fī Tashrīḥ al-ʿurūq ghayr al-ḍawārib* (one maqāla), and *fī Tashrīḥ al-ʿurūq al-ḍawārib* (one maqāla). Ḥunain writes: '… According to Galen, his book *fī 'l-ʿUrūq* is one treatise in which he describes the arteries and veins. He wrote it for students and addressed it to Antisthenes. The Alexandrians, however, divided it into two treatises: one *fī 'l-ʿUrūq ghayr al-ḍawārib*, and one *fī 'l-ʿUrūq al-ḍawārib*. Except for certain similarities between the

---

bern (Berlin, 1930). An English translation is a desideratum even eighty odd years after its appearance. For a critique of Meyerhof, see Joep Lameer, "From Alexandria to Baghdad: Reflections on the Genesis of a Problematical Tradition," in Remke Kruk and Gerhard Endress (eds.), *The Ancient Tradition in Christian and Islamic Hellenism. Studies on the transmission of Greek philosophy and sciences dedicated to H.J. Drossaart Lulofs on his ninetieth birthday* (= CNWS *Publications* 50), (Leiden, 1997), 181-191. Nonetheless, Meyerhof's itinerary remains a useful scheme; see, for example Dimitri Gutas, "Paul the Persian on the classification of the parts of Aristotle's philosophy: a milestone between Alexandria and Baġdâd," *Der Islam* 60 (1983), 231-267; John W. Watt, "The Syriac Aristotle between Alexandria and Baghdad," *Journal for Late Antique Religion & Culture* 7 (2013), published online at http://www.cf.ac.uk/share/research/centres/clarc/jlarc/contents/volume-7-2013.html, with link to PDF article. Last accessed June 2, 2014.

6 Albert Z. Iskandar, "Bibliographical Studies in Medical and Scientific Arabic Works: Galen's "fī ʿAmal al-tashrīḥ" (On Anatomical Procedures), the Alexandrian Book Entitled "fī'l-Tashrīḥ ilā 'l-mutaʿallimīn"(On Anatomy for Students), and Rhazes' "al-Kāfī fī'l-ṭibb" (The Sufficient Book on Medicine)," *Oriens* 25 (1976), 133-147.

> closing passage of maqāla XIII (*fī 'Amal al-tashrīḥ*) and that of the *Tashrīḥ al-'urūq al-ḍawārib* the texts in question are quite different.[7]

Iskandar illustrates these differences by citing some passages from both Galen (in Arabic translation) and the summary. One can only second Iskandar's call, made some forty years ago, for editions—and studies—of the two texts. In particular, we call attention to the two examples displayed on pages 143-144 of his paper, which may possibly indicate some difference in understanding the cardiovascular system. Since late antiquity, "Galenists" have differed on the proper understanding. In a lengthy paper on this subject, Jeremy Bylebyl and Walter Pagel observe:

> This difference over the source of the arterial blood in the pulmonary veins probably reflects a more general difference between Galen and many of the later Galenists concerning the source of arterial blood. In Galen's view the blood of the arteries could be derived from the veins through peripheral anastomoses, rather than from the left ventricle of the heart, and still be perfectly good arterial blood. This was because the arteries selectively take up only the lightest portions of the venous blood, and it was this difference in consistency that above all distinguished the two kinds of blood. The later Galenists, by contrast, tended to think of arterial blood as a unique product of the left cardiac ventricle, just as venous blood is of the liver.[8]

By "later Galenists" the authors intend mostly late medieval and renaissance scientists; but they did not look at the summaries. The passages cited by Iskandar are not sufficient for any further discussion here, but they do raise the possibility of some difference between the summaries and Galen which deserves further investigation.

A summary of Galen's book *On Temperament* (*fī al-mizāj*) is found on ff. 154v-167r of MS 113 (item 2222) of the Daiber collection, now located in Tokyo.[9] It bears the title *Jumal wa-jawāmi' al-Iskandar fī ta'arruf al-mizāj*; however, the name al-Iskandar has been added above the line, in what seems to be a later hand. The list of titles found on f. 1v of the manuscript informs us

---

7 Ibid., 140-141.

8 Jerome J. Bylebyl and Walter Pagel, "The chequered career of Galen's doctrine on the pulmonary veins," *Medical history* 15 (1971), 211-229, at p. 211.

9 The description is accessible online at: http://ricasdb.ioc.u-tokyo.ac.jp/daiber/fra_daiber_I_II.php?vol=2&ms=Ms.113&txtno=2222; images are available as well at the same website, as well as at al-mostafa.com. Both last accessed June 2, 2014.

that this work derives from Hippocrates (*min kalām Abūqrāṭ*). Fortunately Professor Daiber provides a very detailed description of the text; in particular, he compared it with all known epitomes of this work, and it differs from them all. Though the copyist may have assumed that this is a copy of the Alexandrian summary, and therefore added the name al-Iskandar, Daiber's comparison with the citations in Dietrich's *Medicinalia* reveals that the two are not the same.[10] Daiber's suggestion, "Our text may be an independent Arabic adaptation of Galenic themes" is right on the mark; the Alexandrian *jawāmiʿ* were likely the most important of these adaptations, but certainly not the only ones. We thought it prudent to check the text against the Hebrew translation of the Alexandrian summary, seeing that our work on *On Critical Days* demonstrates conclusively that the Hebrew version is not translated from any extant Arabic text. Comparison with MS Vienna shows that the two are not related at all; Daiber's manuscript has been drastically shortened, even relative to the Alexandrian summary. Daiber adds that his text has no relationship to the redactions (*talkhīṣāt*) of Ibn Rushd. Those belong to a much later period; we will have something to say about them below.

More recently, Peter Pormann has taken a close look at the summary of *On the Sects for Beginners.*[11] Pormann states, "By looking at an individual text and describing it in great detail, one can dispel some of the misconceptions which scholars have formed of these 'summaries'."[12] He correctly observes that the summaries differ from each other in their approach to the Galenic text, and, therefore, what one learns about a single summary cannot be automatically applied to all the rest. With this in mind, Pormann sets out to examine the text he has chosen and its relationship to Galen's original, as well its relationship to other late antique texts, including commentaries and abridgments by Yaḥyā al-Naḥwī ("John the Grammarian"). This is very much the path we have chosen with regard to *On Critical Days*. However, Pormann's ultimate goals differ: he is mainly interested in learning how medicine was taught in Alexandria and how philosophy and medicine influenced each other.

We will briefly review some of Pormann's principal findings. The summaries exhibit "a strange mixture of further division and subdivision of as-

10 Albert Dietrich, *Medicinalia Arabica: Studien uber arabische medizinische Handschriften in turkischen und syrischen Bibliotheken* (Göttingen, 1966), 36.

11 Peter E. Pormann, "The Alexandrian Summary (*Jawāmiʿ*) of Galen's On the Sects for Beginners: Commentary or Abridgment?" in Peter Adamson (ed.), *Philosophy, Science and Exegesis in Greek, Arabic and Latin Commentaries* (London, 2004), 11-33.

12 Ibid., 11.

pects of medicine, not always closely connected with the original…".[13] While nothing of the sort is found in the summaries of *On Critical Days*, most likely because it would not have been perceived to have been needed or useful, we do find complex diareses in the summaries of *On the Elements According to Hippocrates*.[14] Galen's text is paraphrased, the information is organized differently than in the original, and the proportional allocation of space to a given issue also differs from the original: all of these features, which Pormann has found in *On the Sects*, are present in *On Critical Days*, and, indeed, in the other summaries that we have had a chance to inspect in the course of our research.

The summaries occasionally present by way of example information not found in Galen; again, this holds true for *On Critical Days* just as it does for *On the Sects*. However, Pormann finds that the summary of *On the Sects* is actually about ten percent longer than the original (especially if we take into account that Arabic usually uses less words to express an idea than does Greek). Though we have not undertaken to compile statistics, we can say that this feature is not true for *On Critical Days*, which must have seemed to the writers of the summary to have much repetition and superfluous polemics; hence the summary is considerably shorter. On the other hand, the Arabic epitome of *On the Sects* attributed to Yaḥyā al-Naḥwī in British Library, MS Or. Arundel 17 is much shorter than Galen's text or the summary; the same holds for the Yaḥyā's epitome of *On Critical Days*.[15]

In what language were the summaries originally written? Pormann cites earlier scholarship, all of which claims a Greek original, even though no trace of a Greek text has been found, and seems to concur: "In the whole of *Jaw*[*āmiʿ*] *firaq* I have not found any reference which would point to an Arabic or an Islamic context. This, in itself, is of course not sufficient evidence for *Jaw*[*āmiʿ*] *firaq* having been written originally in Greek, but it makes it more probable."[16] *On Critical Days* does have some transcriptions of

13 Ibid., 13.

14 Tzvi Langermann, "Islamic Atomism and the Galenic Tradition," *History of Science* 47 (2009), 277-295, at p. 285.

15 Langermann, "The Astral Connections of Critical Days," 113-115. Yaḥyā's epitome of *On Critical Days* takes up only about five pages in the unique manuscript; however, it is followed by an independent essay which argues that the critical days relate to the lunar phases. Pormann has published separately a lengthy study of Yaḥyā's epitome of *On the Sects*: "Jean le grammarien et le De sectis dans la littérature médicale d'Alexandrie, " in Ivan Garofalo and Amneris Roselli (eds.), *Galenismo e medicina tardoantica: fonti greche, latine e arabe* (Naples, 2003), 197-248.

16 Pormann, "Alexandrian Summary," 26.

Greek words, which does not necessarily prove that the original was written in Greek; but it also has an important hint at a Syriac original, or at least, a Syriac *Vorlage*.[17]

Emilie Savage-Smith begins her close study of a summary on ophthalmology ascribed to Galen with some prudent, cautionary observations concerning the *jawāmiʿ* or summaries: "Occasionally a compiler of the *jawāmiʿ* is named, such as Thābit ibn Qurah (d. 901) or the enigmatic figure known in Arabic as Yaḥyā al-Naḥwī. In most instances, however, the compiler is anonymous and it is uncertain whether the summary was originally made in Greek, Syriac, or Arabic. The statement in a manuscript that a treatise was translated by Ḥunayn ibn Isḥāq is not sufficient evidence, by itself, for maintaining that it was translated from the Greek and that Ḥunayn made the translation, for virtually every manuscript copy of a work claiming a Greek origin has such a statement."[18] Accordingly she will first present a "brief review of the fragility of the evidence for confidently associating any of them with the Alexandrians, and a reminder of the testimony of Ḥunayn ibn Isḥāq as to the existence of Galenic summaries in his day" (this is the text we cited above, in the translation of Max Meyerhof), before proceeding to the examination of the treatise on eye diseases.

Savage-Smith goes on to remind us that Ḥunayn mentions only one summary by name, *On the Therapeutic Method*, and does not associate it with the Alexandrians. Moreover, Ḥunayn tells us that he himself prepared some thirteen summaries; but he also informs us of the form (some tabular, others question and answer) in which they were written, and none of the extant copies of the summaries fits those descriptions. Hence a conundrum: the summaries should be the work of Ḥunayn, but they do not match his description of his own writings. Savage-Smith provides us with what is certainly the most thorough listing of all treatises, and all manuscripts, that may be considered part of the summary genre; there is no call for us to reproduce that here.

Turning now to her text on ophthalmology, Savage-Smith notes that it "consists basically of an enumeration of ninety-one eye diseases and symptoms, intermixed with many Greek terms (in transliteration) and ending with a listing of the parts of the eye with an accompanying diagram of the visual system."[19] We note that the summary of *On Critical Days* also has

---

17 See below, [19].

18 Emilie Savage-Smith, "Galen's lost Ophthalmology and the Summaria Alexandrinorum," *Bulletin of the Institute of Classical Studies* 45 (2002), 121-138, at p. 138.

19 Ibid., 132.

Greek words in transliteration, though no diagrams (diagrams are stressed by Pormann as well). Moreover, since the original of Galen's work on eye diseases is lost, Savage-Smith's basic question differs from our own. She cannot compare the summary with the original; instead, she wishes to explore whether or not it can be determined that the Arabic summary truly represents, even if in summary form, the lost writing of Galen. For this reason her study cannot help us to determine just how and to what extent the summaries are a revision of Galen. Nonetheless, the information that she has amassed is very useful, and we can second her conclusion:

> The attribution in many of the manuscripts containing various Galenic *jawāmiʿ* to the Alexandrians indicates that in the minds of ninth- and tenth-century Islamic physicians Alexandria was associated with the teaching of Galenic medicine, and that for a manuscript to suggest an association with Alexandria was to enhance its authority and possibly authenticity. It also indicates that Alexandria at that time had a reputation for producing summaries of treatises, even though Ḥunayn makes no mention of such summaries. It also implies that Alexandria had a reputation for distinctive didactic methods of presentation, such as tabular presentation or branch-diagramming or possibly question-and-answer. But there is no secure evidence that such techniques actually were a part of the Alexandrian scene.[20]

With all of this in mind—in addition, of course, to the information to be added in the present publication—we must take with caution the report of the tenth-century Andalusian medical writer and historian of medicine, Sulaymān ibn Ḥassān Ibn Juljul, that the group of Alexandrian philosophers who prepared the summaries "did not alter the originals (*wa-lam yughayyiru al-uṣūl*)".[21] As we have seen, the close comparison with the originals (including the Arabic translations of the originals), a project that Ibn Juljul likely did not take upon himself, reveals differences between the original and summary.

Two centuries after Ibn Juljul, Moses Maimonides (d. 1204) prepared two types of abridgements: epitomes (*mukhtaṣarāt*) and his own notebooks (*fuṣūl*). The former covered the same sixteen books that served as the basis of the "Alexandrian" compositions. Maimonides constructed them out

20 Ibid., 138.

21 Ibn Juljul, *Ṭabaqāt al-aṭibbā' wa-'l-hukamā'*, second printing (Beirut, 1985), 51.

of exact quotations from Galen: *ʾataytu fīhā bi-naṣṣ kalām Jālīnūs*.[22] In the beautiful MS Paris BnF heb 1203, which contains three of the epitomes in Hebrew letters, there are a few short comments by Maimonides, as well as one long essay on the synochous fever. These, however, are clearly marked off from Galen by an introductory phrase, *qāla al-muʾallif*.[23] It may have been the awareness that the *jawāmiʿ* make significant alterations to Galen that led Maimonides to prepare these anthologies using only direct quotations.

The *fuṣūl*, or notebooks, by contrast, are a collection of texts, mostly paraphrases, from Galen, with many more additions on the part of Maimonides, some of which are taken from other medical professionals working in Islamicate civilization. The selections are topically arranged, they include materials drawn from the entire Galenic corpus, and the final book (Book XXV) is a systematic critique of Galen.[24]

Maimonides insinuates himself into the Arabic literary tradition with regard to the *fuṣūl*, citing similar works by al-Rāzī, al-Sūsī, and Ibn Māsawayh, and also into the tradition of critiques (*al-shukūk ʿalā Jālīnūs*), mentioning the books of Ibn Zuhr and Ibn Riḍwān.[25] However, he says nothing about a tradition of epitomes, neither the ancient tradition of the Alexandrian summaries, nor those written by or attributed to Ḥunayn or Yaḥyā al-Naḥwī, nor the epitomes produced by his contemporary Ibn Rushd.

Most of the books mentioned by Maimonides are not extant, nor do we possess much of Maimonides' epitomes; the epitomes of Ibn Rushd have not been closely studied, nor have extant notebooks not mentioned by Maimonides, such as the *fuṣūl* of Ibn Sīnā, been subjected to academic scrutiny. In view of this state of affairs, one can offer only a very sketchy historical overview for the continuation of the genre of revised epitomes, in the manner of the Alexandrian *jawāmiʿ*. With all caution, we put forward our suggestion that the notebooks written by Maimonides and others represent the continuation of the *jawāmiʿ*. The literary structure was of course markedly different; moreover; as Maimonides tells us, the notebooks are more personal, containing the information, insights, and observations that

22 Maimonides, *Medical Aphorisms*, 2.

23 Y. Tzvi Langermann, "Maimonides on the Synochous Fever," *Israel Oriental Studies* 13 (1993), 175-98; Gerrit Bos, "Maimonides on Medicinal Measures and Weights," *Aleph* 9 (2009), 255-276.

24 See Bos, "Translator's Introduction," *Medical Aphorisms*, xxii-xxv.

25 The three authors of *fuṣūl* are mentioned in Bos' edition, p. 2. The authors of critiques are mentioned at the beginning of book XXV; see Joseph Schacht and Max Meyerhof, "Maimonides Against Galen: On Philosophy and Cosmogony," *Bulletin of the Faculty of Arts of the University of Egypt* 5 (1937), 53-88 (Arabic section).

one particular physician found to be useful in the course of his career. Yet they were not totally private; they were copied, and indeed enjoyed a wide circulation. Hence it may be the case that, for all the literary differences, the intent was quite similar to that of the *jawāmiʿ*: to provide an abbreviated, accessible version, one that is useful for the author and some readers, based mainly on Galen, but not strictly adhering to his teachings. One may add, the more removed Galen's pronouncements are from medicine, the more severe the criticism.

Maimonides' fellow Cordovan and contemporary Ibn Rushd prepared a number of *talkhīṣāt* or epitomes of Galenic works, or should I say, Galenic topics, which are found, in whole or in part, in two manuscripts at the Escorial, nos. 881 and 884. The Arabic texts have been published twice, first by George Anawati and then again by María Concepción Vázquez de Benito.[26] The latter also published Spanish translations of most of them, and in an introductory essay, conveyed some information about their contents.[27] For example, the *talkhīṣ* of *On Temperament* is an essay on the subject of temperament that draws upon Galen, Aristotle, and the Peripatetics. The very small tract on crisis advances a theory different to Galen's. These epitomes, then, do carry on the tradition of updating Galen, in an even more radical fashion.

---

26 Georges C. Anawati, *Rasāʾil ibn Rushd al-Ṭibbīyah* (Cairo, repr. 2005); María Concepción Vázquez de Benito, *La medicina de Averroes: comentarios a Galeno* (Salamanca, 1987).

27 *Averroes Obra Medica*, trad. María Concepción Vázquez de Benito (Seville and Malaga, 1998, limited edition).

CHAPTER 2

The "Summaries" of *On Critical Days*

Before turning to the text of interest to us, let us summarize briefly our working hypotheses concerning the summaries. Our study of the summaries reveals that they have several unstated goals: (1) to organize the material Galen teaches, in his rambling manner, full of digressions and engagements with other medical authorities, in a more succinct and accessible form; (2) to make some adjustments in medical theory, in line, or so it seems anyway, with developments in the field over the course of the half-millennium (in rough approximation) separating Galen and the summaries; this includes accepting in places views that Galen rejects, and even some outright criticism of Galen.

Though the summaries as a rule avoid Galen's frequent, and frequently long, digressions, some remarks are considered important enough to include even if they perhaps interrupt the flow of the text. An example of this is found in [39], which discusses the authenticity or lack thereof of the books that make up Hippocrates' *On Epidemics*. Perhaps it is not completely accurate to call the omitted passages digressions. They may be for the most part relevant to the issue at hand, but, from the point of view of the summaries, they go into unnecessary detail and intolerable length. An example of this is the examples (perhaps case studies drawn from his practice, but Galen does not say this) of the progress of an illness that take up some two pages of Kühn's text (800-801; Cooper, 150-154).

Despite the efforts of these authors, some of the disorder and repetition of Galen's book is found in the summaries as well. Errors in determining the crisis, the calculation of tetrads, the ways in which the physician can determine which day is critical, are three topics that are discussed more than once, with some repetition. In this respect the version that we refer to for convenience as the Hebrew one (since its Arabic *Vorlage* is not known to be extant) displays a more thorough reorganization. It is a shorter, tighter exposition without repetitions.

Galen begins his book talking about diseases that subside all at once, rather than gradually waning; only after several paragraphs does he tell us that a crisis—when accompanied by indications of a recovery—is a sign that a disease is subsiding . This introductory material is excised in the summaries.

Towards the end of the first book (K 813), Galen tells us that the purpose of this first book is to establish the usefulness of his subject, that is, critical days.

 | DOI 10.1163/9789004282223_003

Needless to say, many other topics are raised, with varying length of exposition. Overall, it seems that the summaries pay more attention to regimen, though Galen does give some space to this topic, especially in the lengthy section dealing with diet from K 884.19 until 886.11 (CG 296-300). Perhaps, then, their practicality consisted not just in drastically shortening Galen's disquisitions, but also in giving more guidance in treating the patient.

The names of Galen's adversaries in the field of medicine (Archigenes, Diocles) are usually left out. An exception is [22 of the Arabic], where Archigenes' counting of critical days is contrasted with that of Galen and Hippocrates. Still, the summary drastically shortens the discussion, as we can see from the following comparison of the two texts:

[22] The critical days after the twentieth day are, according to the adherents of Hippocrates and Galen, the twentieth day, the twenty-fourth, the twenty-seventh, the thirty-first, the thirty-fourth, the thirty-seventh, and the fortieth. But according to the adherents of Archigenes, they are the twenty-first day, the twenty-eighth, the forty-second, the forty-fifth, and the forty-eighth.

CG 178-180 (K 815.17-816.11): Since we have exhausted this, let us take up what we intended, which is to report about the critical days that are after the twentieth day. We find Archigenes and his followers, and Diocles and his followers stating that the twenty-first day is a critical day. And we find Archigenes mentioning that the crisis occurs in the twenty-first day more often than it occurs in the twentieth day. But I do not see the matter thus, nor did Hippocrates. I shall explain this hereafter. The situation in the twenty-seventh day is similar to this, since I think the crisis occurs in it more often than in the twenty-eighth day. However, the group that I referred to shortly before stated that the crisis occurs in it less often. And the thirty-fourth day also has a good power, and the fortieth day is more powerful than it. As for the twenty-fourth day and the thirty-first day, the crisis occurs in them less often than it occurs in those. Fewer than these but also frequent is the thirty-seventh day, such that it is at the boundary between the (class of) days in which crises occur and (that of) the days in which no crisis occurs. And it is for this reason that no crisis is likely to occur in it.

1 Concise Review of the Arabic Summary with Detailed Comments on Some Key Divergences from Galen

[1] announces a classification of critical days into six types; this classification is not found in Galen. [2]-[4] offer a schematic description of good and bad critical days. [5]-[7] discuss the regimens to be given the convalescent, depending on the seriousness of his illness and the possibility of a relapse. Note that this very practical topic is brought up at the beginning of the summaries. [8] lists the various signs of the crisis, specifying their cause within the body: the organ that is expelling, transferring, or receiving the residue or surplus that is the material cause of the disease, or the residue itself. These same symptoms are found by and large in Galen, but not the linkage just described. [9] discusses the difficulty in determining the critical day, and decides that the true crisis is manifested by the convergence of all six signs. Sometimes less than six signs are present; the crisis is then incomplete, though the day on which at least three are present is used for purposes of counting. [10]-[12] are concerned with good and bad critical days, as well as the days on which crisis is never seen to occur. Passage [11] illustrates well the more concise and decisive formulations one finds in the summaries, as opposed to Galen:

[11] The crisis occurs less often on others, and these are the bad days, for example the sixth day. The crisis occurs then for only a few patients. It is a bad crisis, not complete, not clear, unsure of outcome, and not safe from danger.	Cf. CG 136 (K 791.12-16): In the case of the sixth day, however, the illnesses often resolve in it, but they do not resolve like those in the seventh day. This is because the number of illnesses that resolve in the sixth day is less than the number of illnesses that resolve in the seventh day, and the manner of their resolution in the sixth day is different from the manner of their resolution in the seventh day. For the resolution of the illness in the sixth day is neither excellent nor praiseworthy but in most situations it is bad.

[13] takes up the definition of crisis, and the distinction between the concerns of physicians, on the one hand, and rhetoricians and grammarians on the other, in establishing the correct definition. (788.16-789.4) [14] displays the signs of a bad crisis, the signs on the fourth day of a crisis worsening on the sixth day. [15] and [16] arrange the critical days in order of their frequency; this prompts MS Princeton to add here a long marginalium [M1], explaining the rationale behind Galen's system of ordering. This marginalium may be based on K 783.14.

[15], [16] and [M1] constitute a major reassessment on the part of the authors of the summaries of an abstruse and highly theoretical topic; Cooper discusses Galen's treatment in his commentary, pp. 412-3, concluding that "The underlying principle behind this scheme, however, remains opaque." Note that the Hebrew summaries skip over this issue entirely, apparently because it has no practical relevance. The Arabic summaries, however, retain an interest, and [M1] tries to put things in order.

Both Galen and the summaries have three large classes. Galen classifies the critical days according to the swiftness of the illness' resolution: swiftly in class one, progressively less in the other two. The Summaries, on the other hand, arrange the three large classes in descending order of the frequency, that is, the frequency of the crisis falling on that particular day. Galen subdivides his first class into five groups; the Summaries subdivide their first group into four. Here are the groups, and to their right, the critical days that belong to each:

GALEN, *Class I*

I	7, 14
II	9, 11, 20
III	17, 5
IV	4
V	3, 18

SUMMARIES, *Class I*

I	7, 14
II	9, 19, 20
III	17, 5
IV	3, 18

Galen does not subdivide either the second (intermediate) class, nor the third. Here are the days that belong to each: Class II: 12, 16, 19; Class III: 8, 10, 12, 16, 19. The Summaries, for their part, list as intermediate only two days: Class II: 13, 16. The third class is again subdivided into groups:

I	5, 6
II	8, 15
III	12

[17-18] begins the discussion of the beginning of the illness; this is important, since this will tell us when to begin counting towards the fourth day, the seventh day, and so forth. The problem is not easy, as people react differently towards illness, for example, how soon they take to bed. [19] The

onset of the disease can be viewed in two ways: 'by nature', i.e., theoretically, whereby we conclude that the disease began at a certain moment, even though no symptoms are yet present; and empirically. [20] If there is no warning, one must apply theory in order to determine the critical day.

[21] describes the three 'moments' of the crisis, and their use in determining the critical day, when there is some doubt because signs of crisis appear on two consecutive days. Here are the two sets of instructions, the left column from the summaries, the right column from Galen:

[21] There are three moments in which the crisis takes place. One of these is the moment of the fever's paroxysm, the second the moment of evacuation, and the third, the moment or relief from the illness (*takhalluṣ*) [See note 102 to our translation of the passage]. If these moments are present on the same day, we say that that is the critical day. If they take place on two days, then only the day about which the warning day gave warning ought to be called the critical day. If the crisis takes place on two days, then, should most of the critical symptoms be found on the first of them, but only some of them on the second day, then some of the crisis should be given to the second day. But if these symptoms are found altogether on the two days, then the crisis applies to both of them.

Cf. CG 170 (K 810.16-811.9): And let your examining the number of the changing points (lit. the times) of the crisis be in this manner: the[1] changing points of the crisis are three: the first is the beginning of the paroxysm whose arrival indicates a crisis. The second is the beginning of the event in which the crisis occurs via bodily effusion or something else. And the third is the resolution of the crisis. Therefore, the day in which you find two of the changing points of the crisis, is the day more suited to the crisis. And let your examining the interval of the crisis be according to this perspective: examine in which of the two days the interval[2] of the crisis is longer, and that day in which you find the interval[3] of the crisis to be longer is more suited to the crisis. So, if these four signs indicate a single day, then the crisis must belong to this day, and if one of them is substracted, then the crisis likewise belongs to this day. Nevertheless, you must know that the other day has a share in it. So, if the signs that you find in one of the two days are equal (in number) to the signs that you find in the other, then the crisis is shared between them.

1 "changing points"; lit. the times.

2 "interval"; lit. time.

3 "interval"; lit. time.

Overall, the instructions in the summary are a great simplification of Galen's long and detailed treatment of this problem. According to the summaries, if more signs are found on one of the days than on the other, then that day is critical. If the signs are evenly divided between them, then both days are critical. Galen's discussion is found on [K 810.3-811.17]. Noteworthy is Galen's invoking, in the course of his discussion, the classification of odd and even days; even and odd days are important later on [K 820], in determining the day on which the patient will die (if the crisis is bad). Overall, the summaries make far less use in book I of even and odd days; but this is a matter of reorganization, concentrating the discussion of the etiology of critical days in book III. As far as the attitude towards Pythagorean arithmology is concerned, the summaries display a far more positive attitude then does Galen, who in fact mocks it. The shift in attitude towards Pythagoreanism is a striking feature.

[22] exhibits two lists of critical days after day twenty; the one, that of the school of Hippocrates and Galen, the other, that of the school of Archigenes and [23] correlates the critical days to stellar cycles, prompting [M2], a marginalium pointing out that this sort of correlation is found in book II and especially book III, but not here in book I; and indeed the marginalium cites some pertinent information exhibited by "the author of the Summaries" in book III.

Why have the stars been introduced here? On K 817ff. Galen reports Hippocrates' views concerning long-term cycles—seven months, seven years, fourteen years, and twenty-one years. However, no such remark is to be found precisely in the Corpus Hippocraticum. The author of the summaries lists, anonymously, the astral correlates of long-term cycles, then conveys accurately what Hippocrates did record, namely crises falling on days forty, sixty, eighty, and one hundred and twenty. The marginalium is prompted by the reference to the stars, which is out of place in book I.

[24] discusses the exit from the disease; there is nothing to correspond to this passage in Galen's book. [25] summarizes nicely a long disquisition (Cooper 182-186), in which Galen takes up the question of foretelling the course of events, urging the physician to study closely Hippocrates' *Prognosis*, which includes a discussion of weather signs; the physicians should know as well the theory of the pulse. It is not clear from Galen to what extent close study and experience on the part of the physician can substitute for knowledge of Hippocrates' teachings. In the summaries, the matter is clear and concise. There are three requirements for success in prognostication: study of the *Prognosis*, experience in treating patients, and an understanding of the pulse. These three items are mentioned by Galen (K 818.1-7 for study in general and experience, and 818.16 for the pulse.)

[26] introduces the list of signs, [27] lists the signs indicating safety and recovery, while [28] displays the signs of perdition and danger. These three passages have no parallel in Galen. Galen does refer to the signs of recovery, destruction, and danger without specification in [K 819.7-8]. Thus, our text details his general statement. In K 819.7-8 Galen does not generally refer to the signs of recovery, destruction, and danger (this is only in CG 184-5), as he merely refers to the importance of studying the *Prognosis*, and then moves on to a discussion of the signs of concoction, danger, recovery and especially destruction, which is discussed at length (K 819.8-820.5).

[29] discusses the various mishaps that can affect the crisis—meaning, events that interfere with the natural progress of the disease. It is instructive here to take a closer look at the texts, and the sometimes subtle transformations that accompany translation. First, let us display the two expositions in parallel columns:

[29] If the error that befalls the issue of crisis is of a small magnitude, an incomplete crisis is brought about thereby on the seventh day. But if it is of a great magnitude, it is brought about thereby on the ninth day or on the eleventh day. The error may be due to the physician, it may be due to the patient, and it may be due to his family and servants; and it may be due to exterior events, that is, noise, a quarrel with neighbors, and bad news, for example, news of a disturbance or of a fire; or the bringing of sad news concerning family, property, or friend.

Cf. CG 190, 194, 196 (K 822.8-17, 824.1-12): I shall (now) mention these accidents. I maintain that some of them are the patient's own fault, and some are the fault of these our physicians, who think highly of themselves, who think, when one of them calls on the patient that he has not practiced the Art (of medicine) at all, unless he has lifted his garment and tightened his waist, or bandaged him, or applied a hot compress to him, or cauterized him, or bled him, or applied a cupping glass to him, or massaged him, or done something else[4] to him. As many times as they call upon the patient, so many are their mistakes against him. So, if the crisis is prepared to occur in the seventh day, and then he commits a mistake like this against the patient[5] before the seventh day, then it is impossible for the crisis to occur in the seventh day.
I maintain that if a fire occurs in the patient's house, or robbers attack him, or a river engulfs him suddenly, so that the patient is forced to escape—I need not mention what harm will befall him then. Likewise, if he perceives a roof

4 "similar"; add CG 192.
5 "one"; add. add CG 192.

> collapsing, or a wall under[6] which he is, then fear seizes him, and he desires to flee. Or a rainstorm comes, and the house leaks on him, or water falls on his head or on another part of his body, so that it forces him to move away, and he is sleepless and fear or exasperation seizes him. These things also are known to be what harms the patient greatly. Thus also if the neighbors raise a din, and their voices grow louder, or a distressing message reaches the patient, or something similar to this occurs to him, so that the patient is forced to insomnia, then it ruins the accuracy of the doctor's prediction for the patient.

The term "error" reflects different forms of Greek "ἁμαρτάνω", that are used by Galen and that mean in this context, "to go wrong" (see Liddell-Scott, s.v., the meaning listed under A.2; *Greek-English Lexicon* 77). The cause is not necessarily a mistake, though it could refer to a wrong course of action chosen by the doctor; the term refers in general to any unforeseen interference that fouls the natural course of the disease. The Summaries use here forms of the root *kh.ṭ.ʾ*, which also conveys the sense of something going wrong, but leans more towards the notion of error. Ḥunayn, for his part, generally uses forms of the Arabic *ʿ.r.ḍ*, which means "to happen accidentally", reserving *kh.ṭ.ʾ* only for the clear violations on the part of the physician or the patient. (Ḥunayn does uses the substantive *al-khaṭaʾ* in combination with *ʿaraḍa*, which indicates that an error has befallen the case; it seems to one of us, anyway (Langermann), that Ḥunayn is closer to Galen's text, insofar as his wording includes all unforeseen circumstances.)

Galen's biting remarks on pp. 822-3 concerning incompetent physicians, as well as his fairly detailed exposition of the things that are the physicians' responsibility (and cannot be passed off as accidents occurring "from the outside", see K 824-5) are left out of the summary.

[30] addresses the reliability of the prognosis based on the beginning of the crisis, which depends on the type of fever (that is to say, the type of malaria) that the patient is suffering from. Galen goes to great length on the issue of prognostication, urging the doctor to play close attention to the patient's vital signs and averring that it is possible to predict in some, if not most, cases not just the day, but the hour in which the patient will expire. He

6 "under which he is"; "under it" CG 194

knows that some expect the doctor to be a prophet—scrutinizing the medical prognosis more closely and critically than they do augury. The doctor should pay not attention to such slander. Yet Galen testifies [K 834 top] that he has never erred in his judgement. All of this is left out of the summaries.

[31] gives different indications that the patient is safe, and the types of regimen to be given, depending on the diagnosis. [32 and 33] list connections between signs of the disease's ripening and the day on which the crisis will fall. [34] signs off book I.

[35] opens book II with a list of three reasons why there may be differences in the determination of the crisis. The Summaries omit the long discussion with which Galen begins the second book, talking about experience and reason, the need for observations, the references to other works of his and to Hippocrates, and ending up with a reference to the (Platonic) view contrasting the rigid orderliness of the heavens with the seemingly chaotic behavior of earthly processes; once again, the Summaries excise what appear digressions from the main topic of the book. [36] distinguishes between critical days, warning days, and those days that lie in between. [37] Critical days are thought to occur in tetrads—even though often three, rather than four, days separate crises, though the first crisis will not occur before day four. When only three days lie between any subsequent crisis, tetrads are not abandoned; instead two tetrads overlap, so that their sum is seven rather than eight. In that case, the second begins on the last day of the first, so that the sum total of the two tetrads is seven, not eight; here we have 4 + 2nd=7, 7+ 3rd=**11**; 11 + 4th=**14**; 14 +5th =**17**; 17 + 6th =**20**. 7, 11, 14, 17, and 20 are all critical days. There is nothing in Galen's book that corresponds precisely to this passage. Notice, however, that the calculation is designed to fit Galen's remark (K 867.13-14) that day 17 is stronger than day 18, and day 20 is stronger than day 21; the overlaps are arranged so that days 17 and 20 are counted as critical. The passage in the Summaries also recalls K 870.8-ll (CG, p. 274), where Galen quotes Hippocrates' *Prognosis* 20.1-16. Hippocrates says there that "periods" end on days four, seven, eleven, fourteen, seventeen, and twenty. The passages are once again arrayed in a table:

[37] The tetrads of the critical days differ with regard to their number. The first tetrad and the second tetrad overlap (*mawṣulūn*); the second tetrad and the third tetrad	K 867.13-15, CG 268-270: We have shown clearly, from the experiences of Hippocrates, that the seventeenth day is stronger than the eighteenth day, and that the twentieth day is stronger than the twenty-first day. K 870.1-11, CG 274: Hippocrates makes this statement in the *Prognostics*...the crisis of every safe

are counted separately; the third and fourth are consecutive, and the fourth and the fifth also overlap, since the fifth terminates on the seventeenth day. So also do the fifth and sixth overlap.	fever in which trustworthy signs appear will occur on the fourth day or before it…This is the first of their periods; and the second ends on the seventh day, and the third on the eleventh day, and the fourth on the fourteenth day, and the fifth on the seventeenth day, and the sixth on the twentieth day.

Galen mentions the seasons as a factor several times, or the differences between outbreaks from one year to another (especially K 873 for the latter); this is not to be found in the Summaries.

[38] There is consensus concerning the critical days up to day fourteen, after which the medical authorities differ, and their different reckonings are displayed. [39] On the authenticity or lack thereof regarding the various books that make up Hippocrates' *On Epidemics*. Once again, a short sentence in the Summaries takes the place of a very long discussion in Galen's book, beginning at K 874.5, which begins with yet another Galenic disquisition on the need to take into account both experience and reason.

Overall, the first part of book II of Galen reads almost like a running commentary to *On Epidemics*, discussing individual cases, the reasoning behind his views, and so forth. Galen cites extensively from book I of *On Epidemics*, offering his comments along the way. None of this is of interest to the authors of the Summaries, who are interested only in counting critical days. Nonetheless, they do not ignore the question of the authenticity of *On Epidemics* We display in the following table the relevant statements from the Summary and from Galen:

[39] Two of the seven of the books by Hippocrates that are called *On Epidemics* are authentic [*ṣaḥīḥān*], there is no doubt about them; they are the first and the third. There is doubt concerning three of them; they are the second, the fourth, and the sixth [corrected in manuscript from "the seventh"]. Two are fabrications and forgeries; they are the fifth and the seventh.	K 895.15, CG 258: So, because some ascribed Books II, IV, and VI of the *Epidemics* to Hippocrates, and others ascribed them to Thessalos, his son, we will mention (only) a few of the many things he stated in them.

[40] Sometimes the crisis lasts for many days, requiring the physician to turn to other data in order to learn about the affair. [41] Some crises are

well-defined, others are not. [42] Brief generalities concerning the end of diseases, [43] on the termination of chronic illnesses in particular. [44] On "true" criticals (those crises falling on the expected days, such as day four, seven, etc.) and false criticals (those that fall on other days).

[45] Knowledge of critical days is useful for prognostication and for prescribing the proper treatment. [46] Hippocrates used nature as criterion for determining the critical days. [47] discusses the even and odd critical days. [48] Critical days have cycles of four, seven, and twenty days .

[49] The causes of discrepancy—that is, the crisis occurring on a day that was not expected to be critical—are many and varied; four are briefly described here. [50] Elaboration on the fourth cause of error or discrepancy: the patient may exhibit the symptoms of more than one illness, whether it be with regard to the type of fever, type of crisis, and the time of critical days. Clearly this condition will confuse the physician and lead to error in determining when precisely the crisis occurs.

[51] Some days are critical, others are critical and warning, yet others fall between these two. [52] This last classification again appeals to the 'overlapping' tetrads. [53] Cycles of four, seven and twenty days, to which is added [M3], a marginalium that seeks to show that Galen was economizing in his classification. Note that the Arabic summaries preserve some of Galen's rambling style, which leads to much repetition and to returning again and again to the same topic. The Hebrew summaries exhibit a more severe reorganization.

[54] Principles for classification of illnesses. [55] General classification (acute and swift, chronic); [56] illnesses of short duration; [57] range of acuity in illnesses; [58] illnesses that terminate on the fortieth day. These issues are discussed at very great length by Galen in *On Critical Days*, with comparisons between Hippocrates' remarks in different texts and barbs directed at the Sophists who carry on prolonged and pointless arguments about nomenclature. Those disquisitions are not found in the Summaries, which present instead completely new restatements, especially in passages [57]-[58]. In the following table we compare the concise statement of [58] with part of Galen's lengthy discussion (K 894.4-17; CG 310):

[58] Among the illnesses that terminate on the fortieth day, some are those that terminate between the onset of the illness and the completion of fourteen days; others begin when it moves with acute movements during the critical days until after the twentieth [day]; yet others [marginalium: that is, from among the illnesses that are chronic] take on this configuration afterwards. Their termination is either within seven months, or within seven years, or within fourteen years

Therefore, if he had said in the *Prognostics* that the fortieth day was a critical day for acute illnesses, and if he had said in the *Aphorisms* that their crisis occurs in fourteen days, perhaps it is possible for someone to imagine that the matter is indeed as these say, [namely that the crisis of acute illnesses occurs as these say]. So, when he said in the *Prognostics*, on the one hand that the crisis of the acute illnesses will occur in forty days, and he said in the *Aphorisms* on the other that its crisis will occur in fourteen days, then the interpretation of this statement, which is one kind with two conflicting interpretations, is worthy of scorn...We have shown sufficiently that Hippocrates expressly made the fourteenth day the limit of illnesses that are called simply acute, and regarding the acute illnesses occurring from the relapse, (he set the limit) in some cases on the fortieth day, and in other cases the sixtieth day, in view of what is useful for teaching us about them.

[59] Galen's view on acute illnesses. [60] Characteristics of illnesses whose crisis comes on the twentieth day. [61] End book II.

[62] Book III. The third book is concerned mainly with the etiology of critical days, and it is here that we find the most thorough reform of Galen's book by the authors of the Summaries, especially in the Hebrew version, to be discussed below. The main differences between Galen's book, the two versions of the Summaries, and some other late antique or early Islamic sources as well, have already been published in an earlier study.[7] Book III opens with yet another statement of Galen's fundamental approach: the two principles upon which knowledge of critical days is based are experience and reason (or theory). [63] introduces the seven shapes of the moon, in the course of its synodic cycle. Greek names are displayed, transcribed into Arabic characters. But a marginalium [M4] states simply and briefly, "I did not find the Greek names in the text". To which text does the note refer? Obviously not the Summaries, where the Greek names are transcribed.

7 Langermann, "The Astral Connections of Critical Days".

However, the Greek names are not found in Ḥunayn's translation (see GC, p. 324). Thus the student of *On Critical Days* whose notes are in the margins of the Princeton manuscript has obviously compared the Summaries to Galen's book. [64] gives a concise account of the astronomical seasons. [65] The intensity of atmospheric events is connected to the moon's synodic cycle. [66] Reasons for the discrepancy in the lapse of time, from month to month, between the last and first visibility of the moon. [67] The heptads of the synodic cycle are noted once again, as in passage 63, but this time taken with reference to an idealized ecliptic, taking, we presume just as an example, that the moon begins the synodic month in Taurus. The authors are then using the same illustration used by Galen, but in a somewhat different mannner, at K 910.16-911.8.

[68] This section has its own title; structurally it is displayed as an appendix or an independent treatise on the cycles of critical days. There are daily, monthly, and yearly cycles, which have stellar analogues; in the ascending order of the length of the cycle, they are cycles of the moon, sun and Saturn. Galen collated only the solar and lunar cycles; the Summaries have introduced Saturn in order to have a stellar analogue for longer cycles.[8] [69] The onset of the disease is either the visually perceived signs of the illness, or the change in the air that is due to a solar or lunar cycle (and to which an illness can be traced back, at least in some cases?) [70] Anomalies in the critical days may be due to the severity of the illness, or to intervention by the physician, the patient, or the patient's entourage. [71] describes critical days "that fall in between". [72] comprises a more detailed look at these anomalies, and their effect on the way the body moves more swiftly or more slowly to expel the superfluity that is the root cause of the disease. Ideally, the superfluity should be expelled after it has ripened or concocted.

[73] A general rule about the frequency of paroxysms in the different kinds of fever. [74] The Pythagorean theory of numbers and its application to critical days. As one can plainly see from the following comparative table, the Summaries display a dispassionate account. Galen, for his part, heaps much scorn on the Pythagoreans, not all of which has been reproduced in the table:

8 Ibid., 41.

[74] The adherents of Pythagoras claim that numbers are of two kinds. Some are odd, and they are masculine; they are the third, the fifth, the seventh, and the ninth. The crisis comes on the third [day] on account of the strength of the cycle and its compulsion; [on] the fifth, on account of the strength of nature; [on] the seventh, on account of the moon; on the ninth, on account of the error that befalls, when it is great. Others are even, and they are feminine; they are the second, the fourth, the sixth, the eighth, and the tenth.

(Cooper, 356-358): Therefore, the crisis occurs in acute illnesses in the odd days not because all even numbers are feminine and all odd numbers are masculine, since you should not state without qualification that odd numbers are stronger than even...All of their nonsensical talk about the strengths of the numbers is obviously repulsive and ugly. Often, when I think of Pythagoras, I marvel at him since, on the one hand he was a wise man, but on the other, he was content to maintain that the numbers have such power. But now is not the time for nonsensical conversation with him who utters nonsense...the crisis must occur in the third and the fifth days. However, it does not occur in them due to the Moon's period, but it occurs either because the crisis, prepared to come on the fourth day, comes prematurely in the third day due to the severity of the paroxysm; or because nature is tired, and nothing excites it in the fourth day, so it quiets down, and it departs, and it moves to the fifth day...It will come in the ninth day also, because this is midway between two critical days, namely the seventh and the eleventh days...

[75] More on paroxysms, especially those that are continuous or almost so. [76] Explanation why day twenty is also a critical day. [77] On the way weeks ("Galenic" weeks) are conjoined, and [78] on how the quarters are conjoined. [79] Brief recap of the classification of diseases. [80] End of book III.

2 Observations on the Hebrew Summaries

The Hebrew version presents a much more radical reworking of Galen's text, in terms of both organization and content. As far as organization is concerned, we note the subdivision of the three books into smaller sections. Beginning with [9], each of these smaller subdivisions also bears its own title.

As far as content goes, the Hebrew version is even more concise than the Arabic. The latter has eliminated most of Galen's polemics and other digressions, but the authors retain an interest in some theoretical issues, for example, the classification of critical days into three major and several other minor categories. The Hebrew version evinces no interest at all in that complex issue. Here follow some of the key divergences from and additions to Galen's text—and from the extant Arabic as well—after which we give a brief conspectus:

§ [1] The authors discuss the etymology of the term "crisis", which, they aver, derives "from Greek and Syriac". The mentioning of Syriac is a major clue for the puzzling question of the authorship of the Summaries; it indicates that one perhaps need not to look for a Greek *Vorlage*, as we would not expect Greek-speaking Alexandrians to display an interest in Syriac lexicology. They may have been written in Syriac, though there is no evidence as yet for this; or, as seems more likely at the present stage of our knowledge, they were written originally in Arabic by Syriac-speaking Christians, bearers of the Galenic tradition.

§ [25], near the end of book II, and leading into book III, where the causes of critical days, especially the astral causes, are treated extensively. This passage contains a clear and strong statement of the primacy of the heavens as causes: "For the greatest natural principle is that what is in heaven effects what happens on earth, especially the moon, because of all the heavenly bodies it is closest to the earth." Earlier on, in [15], the author had remarked that long-term observations of the critical days confirm the general rule that "nearly everything that belongs to the world of coming into being and passing away follows the course of the moon."

§ At the beginning of book III, Galen discusses extensively the effects or influences of the heavenly bodies. He emphasizes that the most powerful of these is the sun. The moon has discernible effects, to be sure, but these all derive from the sun. The encomium to the sun is omitted in its entirety in the Hebrew summaries, which instead distinguish between the moon and all the other stars. Only the moon is important for the theory of critical days.

[1] Definition, symptoms, and etiology of crises. [2] Crisis less relevant to

chronic illnesses. [3-4] Classification of illnesses, especially into the major categories of chronic and acute.

[5-6] The "motion" of the crisis and the days upon which it falls. [7] Utility of knowledge of crises. A fuller argument is found later on, in [13]. [8] The crisis will occur when the illness reaches its maximum, that is, when the surpluses which are the cause of the illness have concocted, unless something throws nature off course.

[9] The concoction of the illness; along with its description are some practical instructions for the physician to prepare the patient for the crisis by means of proper diet and exercise. More such instructions for the period of the crisis follow in [10]. More on the climax and proper diet is found in [11]. In line with basic Hippocratic theory, the patient should eat as little as possible at the time of the climax or in the case of a particularly severe illness. [12] Signs of the good crisis and the bad one.

[13] Knowledge of crises important for prognostication; as such, it is no less useful than signs derived from nature for other things or, for that matter, from other signs useful for medical prognostication, such as bodily evacuations and pulse. [14] Days of warning and days of observation.

[15] Repeated observation has shown that all sublunar events follow the course of the moon, and the critical days are no exception. The passage goes on to emphasize that—for reasons connected to the moon's cycle of 28 days, presumably—crises falling on days seven or fourteen are the best.

[16] Anomalies in the crisis, i.e., its coming earlier or later than expected. Many factors may be responsible. [17] Sometimes, though, the crisis comes on the proper day, but we miss it because we did not know when to begin counting the days, or other symptoms in the patient have misled us. [18] The different types of crisis: complete, defective, trustworthy, safe, etc.

[19] Book II. The critical days and their classification. The classification of the days in the Hebrew version is much simpler than that found in either Galen or the Arabic text. This is another indication that this version of the summaries was much more practical, avoiding intricate theoretical issues such as the taxonomy of the critical days which do not have any significant application in medical practice. [20] Days on which the crisis does not occur. These are days 15, 16, and 19; they are listed by Galen and the Arabic summaries, in somewhat different classifications, as days on which the crisis rarely occurs. [21] The division into (Galenic) "weeks" and the use of "overlapping days" for this purpose; and the cycles that are composed of these weeks. A most abstruse topic. [22-25] Some references to Hippocrates' *Epidemics*, *Prognostics*, and *Aphorisms*, along with explanations taken over from Galen's text.

[26-32] Book III, which consists of a detailed and critical review of the Pythagorean view that numbers are the causes of critical days, followed by a discussion of the relation of critical days to the heavenly bodies. Galen's position is reviewed critically and from a distance; this section is by no means a mere "summary" of the corresponding sections of Galen's book. A detailed analysis is available in Langermann, "The Astral Connections of Critical Days".

CHAPTER 3

The Arabic Versions of the "Alexandrian Summaries" of Galen's *On Critical Days*

The Arabic version, allegedly rendered into Arabic by Ḥunayn ibn Isḥāq al-ʿIbādī (809-873),[1] of the *Alexandrian Summary* of Galen's *De diebus decretoriis* (*On Critical Days*) is extant in two MSS:

1 Princeton University Library, MS Garrett 1G (olim Garrett 1075), fols. 59v-67v.[2] [see page 31]

The MS is a medical miscellany, the first text, a later addition, is written in *nastaʿlīq*, and texts 2-10 are written in careful and professional partly vocalized medium large *naskh*. The MS has marginal notes (mostly *ḥāshiyah* on the part of the scribe, copied by the same hand, see fol. 42b, 53a). It contains two main parts. The first main part, containing Galen's *De arte parva* was copied in Dhū al-Qaʿdah 1138 H/1726 A.D. (colophon, fol. 40a) by Muḥammad Amīn al-Ḥasanī ibn ʿAbd Allāh al-Tūqātī. The second main part contains two sub-sections: the first sub-section contains *Summaries* of the following Galenic texts: *De crisibus, De diebus decretoriis, De febribus differentiis, De methodo medendi, De sanitati tuenda,* and was copied, according to the colophon on fol. 244b, by ʿUthmān ibn ʿAlī ibn Muḥammad al-Samarqandī in 572 H/1176 A.D. The second sub-section contains *De sectibus, De pulsibus ad tirones, De*

---

1 Cf. MS Princeton 1075 fol. 42a, in the introduction to the summary of Galen's *De crisibus*. However, as Emily Savage-Smith remarks ("Galen's lost ophthalmology and the Summaria Alexandrinorum," p. 121), the statement that it was translated by Ḥunayn is not sufficient evidence by itself that Ḥunayn made the translation, since virtually every manuscript copy of a work claiming a Greek origin has such a statement. That Ḥunayn indeed is the author of at least some of the Arabic translations of the *Alexandrian Summaries* is confirmed by his own statement that in addition to the translation into Syriac of the summary of *De methodo medendi*, he translated 11 more summaries, and that some of these Syriac summaries were translated into Arabic by ʿĪsā ibn Yaḥyā, while others were translated either by Ḥunayn himself, or his nephew Ḥubaysh (Savage-Smith, ibid., pp. 125-126).

2 Cf. Sezgin, *Geschichte des arabischen Schrifttums*, p. 149, no. 13; R. Walzer, "Codex Princetonianus Arabicus 1075," *Bulletin of the History of Medicine 28* (1954), 550-552; Galen, *Über die Arten der Fieber in der arabischen Version des Ḥunain ibn Isḥāq*, ed. and trans. Matthias Werhard, Inaugural-Dissertation Ludwig-Maximilians-Universität (Munich 2004), xxxiv-xxxv; Princeton University Digital Library: http://arks.princeton.edu/ark:/88435/5m60qr96j (permanent link), last accessed June 2, 2014.

 | DOI 10.1163/9789004282223_004

ratione curandi ad Glauconem, and *De elementis ex Hippocratis sententia*.

2 Tehran, Mağlis 6037 [see below]

No foliation or date, *taʿlīq* script, unvowelled, unnumbered, except for the last page (763) which ends with: تمّ جميع الكتاب ولله الحمد والمنّة كما هو أهله. The MS is a medical miscellany, containing the *Alexandrian Summaries* of Galen's *De arte parva, De pulsibus ad tirones, De ratione curandi ad Glauconem, De elementis ex Hippocratis sententia, De temperamentibus, De naturalibus facultatibus, De anatomia ad tirones* (*fi'l-Tashrīḥ lil-mutaʿallimīn*); *De locis affectis* (trans. Ḥunayn ibn Isḥāq); *De pulsu magna, De crisibus, De diebus decretoriis, De febribus differentiis, De methodo mededi,* and *De sanitate tuenda*.

The two versions differ significantly in a number of places, and employ different technical vocabularies (see table below). For this reason we have decided to present a synoptic edition, in parallel columns. The Arabic texts of MSS Tehran and Princeton have been vowelled and provided with other diacritical signs. Mistakes in vocalisation featuring in MS Princeton have been corrected throughout. In our translation we have for the most part followed MS Princeton, which seems to us to be more correct and generally free of mistakes. Significant variants from MS Tehran have been recorded in the notes to the translation, using the siglum T.

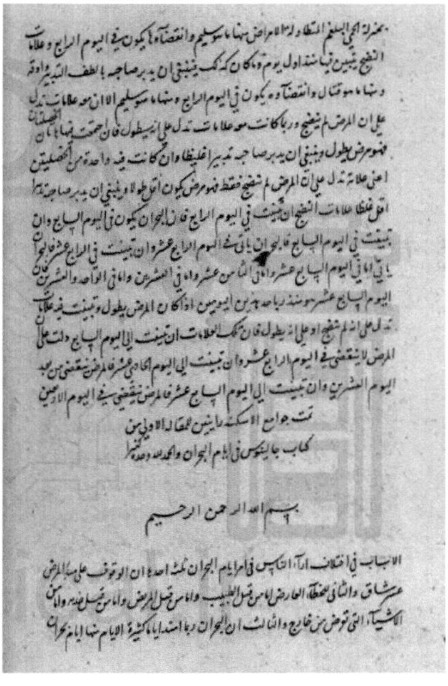

TEHERAN, MAJLIS 6937,
FOL. 228V

Technical vocabularies of the two Arabic versions (selected examples):

Passage	MS Princeton	MS Tehran
2,3,11	بيّن	ظاهر
9	تبيّن	ظهر
9,57,58	انقضى	انحلّ
42	الخروج من المرض	الراحة من الأمراض
42,50	ضروب	أنحاء
43	كان انقضاؤه	انحلّ
43	انقضاء	انحلال
45	سابق العلم	تقدمة معرفة
48	أربعة أربعة	رباعية
48	سبعة سبعة	سابوعية
50	رعاف	فجر الدم
52	حسب	عدّ
55,56,59	وقوع	انحطاط
56	آخر	انتهاء
57,75	انقضى	كان انحلالها
57	طبقات	أقسام
63	المسدّس	ذو الستّ الزوايا
63	تفسير	معنى
63	المقسوم بنصفين	المنصف
63	المربّع	ذو الأربع زوايا
63	المثلّث	ذو الثلاث الزوايا
64	صار فوق رؤوسنا	سامت رؤوسنا
65	تتغيّر تغيّرات	حدث تغايير
68	منزلة	نسبة
73	صنفان	تنقسم قسمان
74	يوما ويوما لا	كلّ ثلاثة أيّام
74	مثال واحد	وتيرة واحدة
78	الأمراض المتريثة	المزمنة

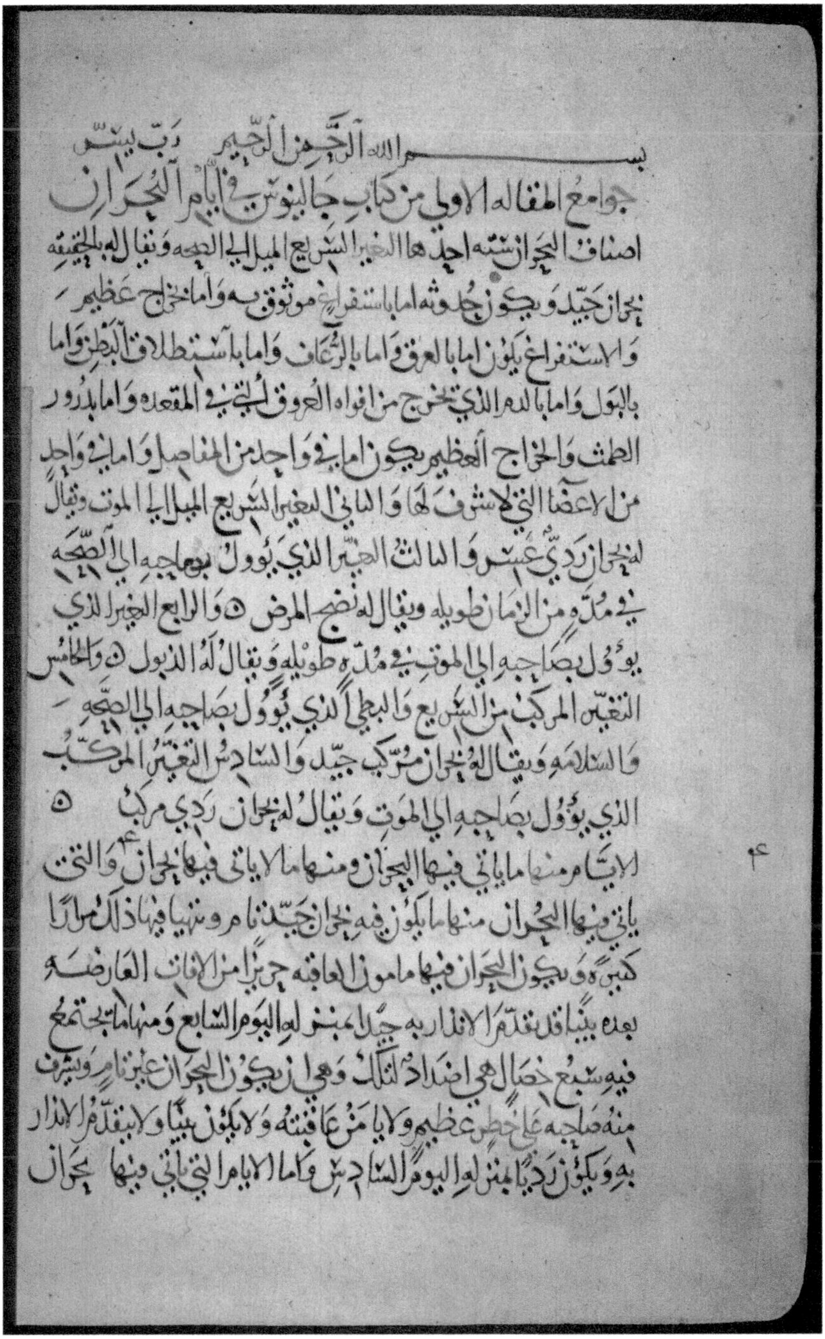

بسم الله الرحمن الرحيم رب يسر

جوامع المقالة الاولى من كتاب جالينوس في ايام البحران

اصناف البحران ستة احدها التغير السريع الميل الى الصحة ويقال له بالحقيقة
بحران جيد ويكون حدوثه اما باستفراغ موثوق به واما بخراج عظيم
والاستفراغ يكون اما بالعرق واما بالرعاف واما باستطلاق البطن واما
بالبول واما بالدم الذي يخرج من افواه العروق التي في المقعدة واما بدرور
الطمث والخراج العظيم يكون اما في واحد من المفاصل واما في واحد
من الاعضاء التي لا شرف لها والثاني التغير السريع الميل الى الموت ويقال
له بحران رديء عسر والثالث التغير الذي يؤول بصاحبه الى الصحة
في مدة من الزمان طويلة ويقال له نضج المرض ٥ والرابع التغير الذي
يؤول بصاحبه الى الموت في مدة طويلة ويقال له الذبول ٥ والخامس
التغير المركب من السريع والبطيء الذي يؤول بصاحبه الى الصحة
والسلامة ويقال له بحران مركب جيد والسادس التغير المركب
الذي يؤول بصاحبه الى الموت ويقال له بحران رديء مركب ٥
الايام منها ما ياتي فيها البحران ومنها ما لا ياتي فيها بحران والتي ٤
ياتي فيها البحران منها ما يكون فيه بحران جيد تام ويتبين فيها ذلك مرارا
كثيرة ويكون البحران فيها مامون العاقبة جيدا من الافات العارضة
بعده بينا قد تقدم الانذار به جيدا منسوبا الى اليوم السابع ومنها ما يجتمع
فيه سبع خصال هي اضداد تلك وهي ان يكون البحران غير تام ويشرف
منه صاحبه على خطر عظيم ولا يامن عاقبته ولا يكون بينا ولا يتقدم الانذار
به ويكون رديا منسوبا الى اليوم السادس واما الايام التي ياتي فيها بحران

PRINCETON UNIVERSITY LIBRARY, ISLAMIC MANUSCRIPTS COLLECTION, GARRETT 1G (OLIM GARRETT 1075), FOL. 59V

1 Princeton MS

[1] بسم الله الرحمن الرحيم رب يسّر

جوامع المقالة الاولى من كتاب جالينوس في أيّام البحران

أصناف البحران ستّة أحدها التغيّر السريع الميل إلى الصحّة ويقال له بالحقيقة بحران جيّد ويكون حدوثه إمّا باستفراغ موثوق به وإمّا بخراج عظيم والستفراغ يكون إمّا بالعرق وإمّا بالرعاف وإمّا باستطلاق البطن وإمّا بالبول وإمّا بالدم الذي يخرج من أفواه العروق التي في المقعدة وإمّا بدرور الطمث والخراج العظيم يكون إمّا في واحد من المفاصل وإمّا في واحد من الأعضاء التي لا شرف لها والثاني التغيّر السريع الميل إلى الموت ويقال له بحران رديء عسر والثالث التغيّر الذي يؤول بصاحبه إلى الصحّة في مدّة من الزمان طويلة ويقال له نضج المرض والرابع التغيّر الذي يؤول بصاحبه إلى الموت في مدّة طويلة يقال له الذبول والخامس التغيّر المركّب من السريع والبطيء الذي يؤول بصاحبه إلى الصحّة والسلامة ويقال له بحران مركّب جيّد والسادس التغيّر المركّب الذي يؤول بصاحبه إلى الموت ويقال له بحران رديء مركّب.

[2] الأيّام منها ما يأتي فيها البحران ومنها ما لا يأتي فيها بحران والتي يأتي فيها بحران منها ما يكون فيه بحران جيّد تامّ وتهيّأ فيها ذلك مرارا كثيرة ويكون البحران فيها مأمون العاقبه حريزًا من الآفات العارضة بعده بيّنا قد تقدّم الإنذار به ‹أنّه يكون› جيّدًا بمنزلة اليوم السابع.

[3] ومنها ما يجتمع فيه سبع خصال هي أضداد لتلك وهي أن يكون البحران غير تامّ ويشرف منه صاحبه على خطر عظيم ولا يأمن عاقبته ولا يكون بيّنًا ولا يتقدّم الإنذار به {60a} ويكون رديئا بمنزلة اليوم السادس وأمّا الأيّام التي ‹لا› يأتي بحران | فبمنزلة اليوم الثاني عشر والسادس عشر.

[4] الأمراض التي تعاود بنكسة يكون بعضها هي أمراض مهلكة قتّالة وهي التي يكون القوّة فيها قد خارت وضعفت وظهرت معها علامات العطب والتلف وبعضها لا يكون قتّالة

لكن ينكس صاحبه فقط وماكان من الأمراض كذلك فهي من قبل أنّ القوّة تكون فيها
[5] صحيحة قوية لا تقتل لأنّ القوّة تكرّ على المرض ثانية فتجاهده حتّى تقهره. | وبعضها يمكن
فيه أن يمنع من العودة والنكسة وهي الأمراض السليمة التي ليس معها أعراض رديئة فإنّ
التدبير اللطيف يبلغ في هذه ما يحتاج إليه من منع المرض من العودة والنكسة.

[6] وينبغي أن يستعمل في الأمراض التي يكون الإنسان منها على ثقة عند انقضائها التدبير
المنعش وهو تدبير الناقهين حتّى يردّ المريض إلى تدبيره الذي كان في وقت صحّته قليلا
قليلا بركوب الخيل والجلوس على الكراسي التي تتحرّك بيكر تحتها وبدخول الحمّام
[7] وشرب الشراب الموافق وأكل الطعام الملائم بمنزلة لحوم الفراريج والسمك الرضراضي. |
وأمّا في الأمراض التي قد سكنت سكونا ليس صاحبه علي ثقة منه فينبغي أن يكون
التدبير مثل تدبير المرضى وذلك أنّه إن كان المرض الذي سكن مرضا يسير المقدار منعه
هذا التدبير من أن يعاود لأنّ الأمراض الليّنة التي ليس معها أعراض خبيثة رديئة قد
يمكن فيها ان تمنع من المعاودة وإن كان المرض عظيم المقدار خبيثا ثم دبّرت المريض بمثل
هذا التدبير الذي كان يتدبّر به في وقت مرضه كان معاودة المرض له معاودة لا يشرف
بها على الخطر وإن دبّرته تدبيرا لا يحرز له فيه كانت نكسته نكسة خطر.

[8] علامات البحران منها ما يكون بسبب العضو الدافع للفضل بمنزلة انجذاب مراقّ
{60b} البطن الى فوق ومنها ما يكون بسبب العضو المؤدّي والمنفذ للفضل | بمنزلة ضيق التنفّس
ومنها ما يكون بسبب العضو القابل للفضل بمنزلة الدموع والصداع واختلاط الذهن
والسبات وثقل الصدغين ووجع الرقبة وخفقان الفؤاد والنافض. ومنها ما يكون السبب
الفضل نفسه بمنزلة اللمع الذي يراه الإنسان وظلمة البصر.

[9] وجود حقيقة أمر الأيّام الباحورية عسر شاقّ وذلك لأنّ انقضاء المرض ممّا يعسر
إدراكه والوقوف عليه ولأنّ البحران ربّما إمتدّ أيّاما كثيرة وإذا كان ذلك فمن الناس من
يقول إنّ اليوم الأوّل هو يوم البحران أعني اليوم الذي فيه إبتدأ تكوّن البحران ومنهم
من يقول إنّ اليوم الثاني هو يوم البحران وهو اليوم الذي يتبيّن فيه أكثر وقت البحران

ومنهم من يقول إنّ اليوم الثالث هو يوم البحران وهو اليوم الذي فيه ينقضي المرض. يوم البحران بالحقيقة هو اليوم الذي يجتمع فيه جميع أعلام البحران وأقلّ منه في عدد أيّام البحران الذي تنقص فيه علامات البحران علامة او علامتين واليوم الذي يميل فيه المرض مثلا لا يستتمّ فيه البحران هو اليوم الذي يكون فيه من علامات البحران وتنقص منها ثلاثة.

[10] الأيّام الباحورية منها ما يكون فيه البحران أكثر وهي أيّام جياد بمنزلة اليوم السابع فإنّ هذا اليوم يأتي ‹فيه› البحران في كثير من المرضى ويكون بحرانه جيّدا تامًّا مأمون العاقبة سليمًا من الخطر قد تقدّم الإنذار به وذلك أنّ اليوم الرابع ينذر بتغيّر يحدث فيه إمّا في النضج الذي يتبيّن في البول أو في النفث أو في البراز وإمّا في الفعل يعني في الشهوة والحسّ والعقل والنوم.

[11] ومنها ما يكون فيه البحران أقلّ وهي أيّام رديئة بمنزلة اليوم السادس فإنّ هذا إنّما يأتي فيه البحران قليلا من المرضى ويكون بحرانه رديئًا وغير تامّ ولا بيّنًا ولا مأمون العاقبة ولا سليمًا من الخطر.

[12] {61a} ومنها ما لا يكون فيه بحران بمنزلة اليوم | الثاني عشر والسادس عشر.

[13] بعض الناس يسمّي كل تغيّر يحدث في المرض دفعة بحرانا وبعضهم إنّما يسمّي بحرانا التغيّر الذي يكون إلى السلامة وبعضهم يسمّي بحرانا ما يتقدّم الانفصال من إضطراب. خاصّة الأطبّاء إن يكون بحثهم عن الأمور أنفسها وخاصّة أصحاب الجدل إن يبحثوا عن صحّة أسمائها وإجراها مجاريها وخاصّة أصحاب إقامة لغة اليونانيين وأصحاب الروطوريقى وهي الصناعة التي تلتمس الإقناع والبحث عن الأسماء التي قد جرت بها العادة والأسماء الغريبة.

[14] إذا كان البحران الذي يقع في اليوم السادس يميل إلى الحال الأردى يعرض قبله في اليوم الرابع صغر نفس وبرد ورعشة وخور القوّة وعرق غير مستو في البدن واستفراغ أشياء لم تنضج.

[15] الأيّام الباحورية منها ما لا يزال البحران يأتي فيها دائمًا ومنها ما لا يكاد يأتي فيه البحران إلّا في الندرة ومنها ما حالها في ذلك حال وسط فأمّا الأيّام التي يكون البحران فيها دائمًا فمنها ما هي في الطبقة الأولى من طبقات أيّام البحران بمنزلة اليوم السابع واليوم الرابع عشر ومنها في الطبقة الثانية بمنزلة اليوم التاسع والتاسع عشر والعشرين ومنها في الطبقة الثالثة بمنزلة اليوم السابع عشر واليوم الخامس ومنها في الطبقة الرابعة بمنزلة اليوم الرابع والثالث والثامن عشر .

[16] وأمّا الأيّام التي يأتي فيها البحران في الندرة فمنها أيضا ما هو في الطبقة الأولى بمنزلة اليوم الخامس والسادس ومنها ما في الطبقة الثانية بمنزلة اليوم الثامن واليوم الخامس عشر ومنها في الطبقة الثالثة بمنزلة اليوم الثاني عشر . وأمّا الأيّام التي حالها حال وسط بين هذه فذلك بمنزلة اليوم الثاث عشر واليوم السادس عشر .

[M1] |(في الهامش:٣ حاشية له أولاها بالندور ما جعله في الطبقة الثالثة ويمثّل عليه بالثاني عشر وذلك خلاف بطبيعة الأيّام التي يكون فيها | البحران دائمًا فإنّه جعل الطبقة الأولى منها أولاها بذلك ويدلّك على ما قلت إنّ جالينوس قال إنّي إلى الغاية | ما رأيت قطّ البحران في الثاني عشر وأمّا السادس وهو ممّا جعله في الطبقة الأولى ممّا يندر فيه | البحران فقد ذكر حدوث البحران الرديء فيه كثيرا وإنّما رتّبت كذلك لأنّه جعل الطبقة الأولى | من التي يأتي فيها البحران في الندرة هو الذي يلي آخر طبقات التي يوجد فيها البحران دائمًا فيكون أكثر| النادرة وجودا وجعل آخر طبقات النادرة الوجود أقلّها وجودا فصارت جميع الأيّام البحرانية | الدائمة الوجود والنادرة الوجود مرتّبة بذلك على حيث الأكثر وجودا ويكون الأولى بالدوام | أوّل؟ الجملة ‹و› الأولى بالندور آخر الجملة) .

[17] {61B} مبدأ المرض عند بعض الناس | هو وقت الإحساس بالأذى وعند بعضهم هو مبدأ إلقاء الإنسان نفسه والناس في هذا الإلقاء مختلفون فمنهم من يلقي نفسه قبل أن يكون المرض لخوره وضعف نفسه ومنهم من يفعل ذلك بعد كون المرض لشدّة نفسه وجودة صبره واحتماله ومنهم من تمنعه أشغاله بأمر دنياه من أن يلقي نفسه فلا يلقيها إلّا في آخر

الأمر وعند بعض الناس مبدأ المرض هو الوقت الذي يحسّ فيه الإنسلن مبدأ أضرار المرض به.

[18] المرضى منهم من يعرض له المرض دفعة من غير أن تتقدّم ذلك علامات تدلّ عليه ومنهم من لا يعرض له المرض دفعة لكن بعد ما ينالهم الأذى ويحدث بهم أعراض المرض فيكون أوّل ما ينالهم الأذى ثمّ يبتدئ بهم الحمّى بعد ذلك.

[19] مبدأ المرض على ضربين إمّا بحسب الطبيعة وهو المبدأ الذي يقول إنّه يبين بالقياس وإمّا بحسب الحسّ وهو الذي يعرف وعليه ينبغي أن يعمل.

[20] متى كان البحران في يومين ولم يكن تقدّمه يوم ينذر به فينبغي أن يستخرج معرفة اليوم الذي هو يوم البحران من قياس الأدوار ومن طبيعة اليوم ومن عدد الأيّام الباحورية ومن وقت البحران.

[21] الأوقات التي يكون فيها البحران ثلثة أحدها وقت نوبة الحمّى والثاني وقت الاستفراغ والثالث وقت التخلّص من المرض وهذه الثلثة الأوقات إن حضرت في يوم واحد قلنا إنّ ذلك اليوم يوم بحران وإن كانت في يومين فليس ينبغي أن يسمّى يوم البحران إلّا اليوم الذي أنذر به اليوم المنذر وإذا كان البحران في يومين إن وجد أكثر الأعراض الباحورية في اليوم الأوّل منها ووجد شيء منها في اليوم الثاني فينبغي أن يعطى اليوم الثاني جزء من البحران فإن وجدت تلك الأعراض في اليومين عامّة فالبحران عامّ لهما جميعا.

[22] {62a} أيّام البحران التي بعد يوم العشرين هي عند أصحاب بقراط | وجالينوس يوم العشرين والرابع والعشرين والسابع والعشرين والواحد والثالثين والرابع والثالثين والسابع والثالثين والأربعين وهي عند أصحاب ارخيجانس يوم الواحد والعشرين والثامن والعشرين والثاني والأربعين والخامس والأربعين والثامن والأربعين.

[23] من أدوار الكواكب ثلثة أدوار هي نظائر أعني دور القمر ودور الشمس ودور زحل وذكر بقراط من أيّام البحران يوم والأربعين ويوم الستّين ويوم الثمانين ويوم المائة والعشرين.

[M2] |(في الهامش: في النصّ[١] في هذه المقالة | ولا عند ما ذكر الكواكب | في الثالثة ذكر زحل واج. . . | مما أخذه صاحب الجوا‹مع›| من البروج هاهنى في(؟)| المقالة الثالثة | قال صاحب الجوامع بعد. . . | في المقالة الثالثة منزل‹ة›| الأربعة عشر إذا قيس ب ‹دور ؟›| القمر وكان على قطر . . . | بمنزلة الستّة الأشه‹ر›| إذا قيست بدور الشم‹س›| ومنزلة الأربعة عشرس‹نة›| إذا قيست بدور زحل) .

[24] الخروج من المرض يكون مع جهاد قوي شديد إلى اليوم الرابع عشر ومع جهاد معتدل قصد إلى يوم الأربعين ولا يكون مع الجهاد إلّا في الندرة فيما بعد الأربعين في الأمراض التي إنّما يكون انقضاؤها على جهة المجاوزة وهي التي يمتدّ فيها البحران إلى ثلثة أيّام.

[25] قال جالينوس إنّه ينبغي لمن أراد أن يتقدّم فيعرف يوم البحران أن يكون عالما بتقدمة المعرفة التي لبقراط وأن يكون قد جرّب واحتنك في مزاولة المرضى بالفعل وأن يكون قد يعلم أمر نبض العروق وأحك‹ا›مه.

[26] العلامت منها ما يدلّ على النجاة والسلامة ومنها ما يدلّ على العطب والتلف ومنها

[27] ما يدلّ على الخطر ومنها ما يدلّ على نضج المرض | فالعلامات الدالّة على السلامة هي أن تكون القوّة قوية والتنفّس سهلا والمريض خفيف البدن والنبض حسنا جيّدا.

[28] والعلامات الدالّة على التلف هي سوء التنفّس وثقل البدن ورداة النبض فأمّا علاملت الخطر فبمنزلة العرق البارد وأمّا علامات النضج فبمنزلة البول النضيج.

[29] {62B} الخطأ العارض في أمر المرضى إن كان يسير المقدار حدث بسببه في يوم السابع | بحران غير تامّ وإن كان عظيم المقدار حدث عنه ذلك في اليوم التاسع أو في اليوم الحادي عشر. الخطأ يكون إمّا من قبل الطبيب وإمّا من قبل المريض وإمّا من قبل خواصّه وخدمه وإمّا من قبل الاشياء التي تعرض من خارج بمنزلة الصياح والخصومة في الجيران والأخبار المؤذية مثل خبر شغب أو حريق أو ورود خبر يغمّ من أهل أو مال أو صديق. البحران في

١ النصّ: emendation eds الفصّ P

الأمراض التي تؤول إلى السلامة يتأخّر وفي الأمراض القتّالة يتقدّم فيكون إمّا في اليوم الخامس إذا كان المرض حادًّا ونوائبه في أيّام أفراد والخطأ في أمر المريض عظيم وإمّا في اليوم السادس إذا كان الأمر على ضدّ ذلك.

[30] من الأمراض ما يمكننا أن نتعرّف منذ أوّل الأمر نوع كلّ واحد وآخر ما ينتهي إليه بمنزلة حمّى الغبّ التي تتبيّن فيها علامات النضج ويكون انقضاؤها في اليوم الرابع ومنها ما لا يمكن أن يقف فيها على معرفة شيء من هذين بمنزلة الحمّى الغبّ إذا كانت حمّيان وكانت أيّامها الأوّل قد تبيّنت فيها علامات تدلّ على أنّ المرض لم ينضج ومنها ما يعرف نوعها ولا يعرف آخر ما ينتهي إليه بمنزلة حمّى البلغم.

[31] الأمراض منها ما هو سليم وانقضاؤه يكون في اليوم الرابع وعلامات النضج يتبيّن فيه منذ أوّل يوم وما يكون كذلك فينبغي أن يدبّر صاحبه بألطف التدبير وأدقّه ومنها ما هو قتّال وانقضاؤها يكون في اليوم الرابع ومنها ما هو سليم إلّا أنّ معه علامات تدلّ على أنّ المرض لم ينضج وربّما كانت معه علامات تدلّ على أنّه سيطول فإن اجتمعت فيه الخصلتان فهو مرض يطول وينبغي أن يدبّر صاحبه تدبيرا غليظا وإن كانت فيه واحدة منهما أعني علامة تدلّ على أنّ المرض لم ينضج فقط فهو مرض يكون طوله | {63A} أقلّ وينبغي أن يدبّر صاحبه تدبيرا أقلّ غلظا.

[32] علامات النضج إن تبيّنت في اليوم الرابع فالبحران يكون في اليوم السابع وإن تبيّنت في اليوم السابع فالبحران يأتي في اليوم الرابع عشر وإن تبيّنت في اليوم الرابع عشر فالبحران يأتي إمّا في السابع عشر وإمّا في الثامن عشر وإمّا في العشرين وإمّا في الواحد والعشرين فإنّ اليوم السابع عشر ينذر بواحد من هذه الثلثة الأيّام.

[33] إذا كان المرض يطول وتبيّنت فيه علامات تدلّ على أنّه لم ينضج أو على أنّه يطول فإنّ تلك العلامات إن تبيّنت إلى اليوم السابع دلّت على أنّ المرض ينقضي في اليوم الرابع عشر وإن تبيّنت في اليوم الحادي عشر فالمرض ينقضي من بعد اليوم العشرين وإن تبيّنت في اليوم السابع عشر فالمرض ينقضي في اليوم الأربعين.

[34] تمّت جوامع المقالة الأولى من كتاب جالينوس في أيّام البحران والحمد لله وصلواته على نبيّه محمّد وآله الطاهرين.

[35] {63B} | بسم الله الرحمن الرحيم

جوامع المقالة الثانية من كتاب جالينوس في أيّام البحران السبب في اختلاف الناس في أمر البحران ثلثة[٢] أشياء أحدها أنّ الوقوف على مبدأ المرض عسر شاقّ الثاني أنّ الخطأ يعرض إمّا من الطبيب وإمّا من المريض والثالث أنّ البحران ربّما امتدّ أيّاما كثيرة.

[36] الأيّام منها أيّام بحران ومنها أيّام إنذار ومنها أيّام واقعة في الوسط أمّا أيّام البحران الصحيحة فالرابع والسابع والحادي عشر والرابع عشر والسابع عشر والعشرون وأمّا الأيّام التي تنذر بأيّام البحران فالرابع والحادي عشر والرابع عشر فأمّا الأيّام الواقعة في الوسط فالثالث والخامس والسادس والثالث عشر والخامس عشر.

[37] أرابيع أيّام البحران يختلف عددها فالرابوع الأوّل والرابوع الثاني يعدّان موصولين والرابوع الثاني مع الرابوع الثالث يعدّان متفرّقين والثالث والرابع موصولين والرابع والخامس أيضا موصولين لأنّه ينتهي الخامس في اليوم السابع عشر وكذلك أيضا الخامس والسادس موصولين.

[38] والقدماء كلّهم اتّفقوا على أيّام البحران إلى اليوم الرابع عشر فأمّا في الأيّام التي بعدها فقد اختلفوا وذلك أنّ قوما منهم يزعمون أنّ أيّام البحران من بعد الرابع عشر هي اليوم السابع عشر واليوم العشرون واليوم الرابع والعشرون واليوم السابع والعشرون واليوم الواحد والثالثون واليوم الرابع والثالثون واليوم الأربعون واليوم الستّون واليوم الثمانون واليوم المائة والعشرون. وقوم آخر يزعمون أنّها اليوم الثامن عشر والواحد والعشرون والخامس والعشرون والثامن {64A} | والعشرون والإثنان والثلثون والخامس والثلثون والإثنان

---

٢ حاشية له: ثلاثة أشياء عسر الوقوف ‹عليها› مبدأ المرض وعروض الخطأ وامتداد البحران P[1]

والأربعون والثامن والأربعون.

[39] كتب أبقراط المسمّاة أبيديميا سبعة منها كتابان صحيحان لا شكّ في أمرهما وهما الأوّل والثالث وثلثة يشكّ في أمرها وهي الثاني والرابع والسابع[٣] واثنان مفتعلان مزوّران وهما الخامس والسابع.

[40] إذا كانت الأمراض أمراضا يمتدّ فيها البحران إلى أيّام كثيرة فينبغي لنا أن نتعرّف أمر البحران من ابتداء المرض ومن اليوم المنذر بالبحران ومن حركات نوائب المرض.

[41] البحرانات منها ما هي محدودة وهي التي تكون وتنقضي في يوم واحد ومنها غير محدودة وهي التي تمتدّ إلى أيّام كثيرة.

[42] الخروج من المرض يكون على ثلثة ضروب إمّا بالنضج إذا فني الشيء الفاعل للمرض على طول الزمان وإمّا بالاستفراغ إذا اندفع الشيء الفاعل للمرض إلى خارج كلّه وإمّا بخراج أو قرحة اذا اندفع ذلك الشيء إلى عضو غير شريف.

[43] الأمراض المزمنة منها ما يكون انقضاؤه بالنضج والتحلّل ومنها ما يكون انقضاؤه دفعة وذلك عندما يتحرّك المرض في آخر الأمر حركة حادّة وأيضا من الأمراض المزمنة ما يمتدّ البحران أيّاما كثيرة ومنها ما يبتدئ وينقضي بحرانه في يوم واحد.

[44] طبيعة أيّام البحران طبيعتان وذاك أنّ منها باحورية حقّ ومنها باحورية زور أمّا الباحورية الحقّ فتسمّى باحورية بالطبع وهي اليوم الرابع والسابع والرابع عشر والعشرون والباحورية الزور هي الثالث والخامس والتاسع والثالث عشر.

[45] المنفعة في العلم بأيّام البحران منفعتان وذلك أنّها ينفع في سابق[٤] العلم بالبحران لأنّا إنّما نعرف البحرانات من الآثار والدلائل التي ينذر بها وينفع في تقدير الغذاء وذلك أنّا إن {64B} عرفنا اليوم الذي فيه يكون انقضاء المرض وقدّرنا الغذاء بحسب ذلك.

[46] وقد ذكر أبقراط الأيّام الباحورية بالطبع وهي أيّام البحران الحقّ والأيّام الواقعة فيما بين

---

٣ والسابع: السادس P1

٤ سابق: P1 سائر P

أيّام البحران الحقّ وذاك أنّه ذكر تلك في كتاب الفصول وفي كتاب تقدمة المعرفة وذكر في المقالة الأولى من كتاب أبيذيميا تلك التي هي أيّام بحران بالطبع والأيّام الواقعة فيما بينها.

[47] وهذه الأيّام الواقعة فيما بينها منها ما تقع في الأزواج ومنها ما تقع في الأفراد أمّا التي تقع في الأزواج فالسادس والثامن والعاشر والعشرون والثامن والعشرون وأمّا التي تقع في الأفراد فالثالث والخامس والتاسع.

[48] أدوار أيّام البحران منها ما يكون في أربعة أربعة ومنها ما يكون في سبعة سبعة ومنها ما يكون في عشرين عشرين أمّا التي تكون في الأرابيع فالأيّام التي تبلغ إلى اليوم العشرين وأمّا التي تكون في الأسابيع فالأيّام التي من العشرين إلى الرابع والثلثين وأمّا التي تكون في العشرينات فالأيّام التي من الأربعين إلى الستّين.

[49] أسباب الاختلاف في أمر أيّام البحران كثيرة أحدها الجهل بأمر طبيعتي أيّام البحران أعني التي هي أيّام بحران بالطبع والتي هي زور والثاني أن يقصتر الطالب لها على طلبها بالكلام والقياس دون التجارب والثالث أن يكون الإنسان متى رأى يوما من الأيّام قد وقع فيه بحران مرّة واحدة قضى عليه بأنه من أيّام البحران ولم يتنظّر حتّى ينظر هل يكون فيه أيضا بحران مرار أخر أم لا والرابع أن يكون الإنسان لا يعلم أنّ أيّام البحران وضروب البحرانات قد تكون وافدة كالأمراض الوافدة الوفود يكون في الأمراض وفي ضروب البحرانات وفي أيّام البحران.

[50] أمّا في الأمراض فإنّ في بعض الأوقات تكون حمّيات محرقة وفي بعضها حمّيات غبّ وفي بعضها حمّيات ربع وأمّا في ضروب البحران فإنّ البحرانات تكون في بعض الأوقات {65A} بالرعاف وفي بعضها بالعرق وفي بعضها بالقيء | وأمّا في أيّام البحران فإنّ منها ما يكون في هذا الوقت في اليوم السابع ومنها ما يكون في وقت آخر في اليوم العاشر ومنها في وقت آخر في اليوم الحادي عشر.

[51] الأيّام منها باحورية فقط وهي اليوم السابع والرابع عشر والعشرون ومنها باحورية

منذرة معا وهي اليوم الرابع والحادي عشر والسابع عشر ومنها واقعة في الوسط وهي الثالث والخامس والثالث عشر.

[52] مقايسة الأيّام تكون على هذا النحو أمّا الأيّام التي قبل يوم العشرين فالأسبوعان الأوّلان منها يحسبان حسابا يفرق فيها بين الأسبوع الأوّل والثاني والأسبوع الثالث يحسب مع الأسبوع الثاني حسابا يوصل فيه هذا بذاك وأمّا الأيّام التي من بعد العشرين فالأسبوعان الأوّلان منها يحسبان أيضا حساب تفريق وينتهيان في اليوم الرابع والثالثين والأسبوع الثالث يوصل بالأسبوع الثاني وينتهي في يوم الأربعين.

[53] الأدوار ثلثة فواحدة منها دور النصف وهو دور الأرابيع لأنّ الأربعة إذا ضعفت صارت منها الثمانية والإثنا عشر والستّة عشر والآخر دور تامّ وهو دور الأسابيع لأنّ السبعة إذا أضعفت صار منها الأربعة عشر والواحد والعشرين والثمانية والعشرين والخمسة والثلثين والإثنين والأربعين. والدور الثالث دور أتمّ من هذا وهو دور العشرينات لأنّ العشرين إذا أضعفت صارت منها أربعين وستّين وثمانين ومائة وعشرين.

[M3] |(في الهامش: في النصّ فينبغي إذن أن نقسم قسمة لا يلزمنا من قبلها أن نضيف الأجزاء المتباينة بعضها إلى بعض وذلك يكون إذا قسمنا ذلك الشيء الذي ينسب إلى الكمّية الى اجزاء كبار ولا يتجاوز في القسمة الحدّ حتّى تكثر الاجزاء جدّا فتتجاوز المقدار الذي يصلح للتعليم.)

[54] ينبغي أن تجعل قسمة الأمراض قسمة لا تكون بحسب الأيّام الباحورية وإلّا صارت إلى ما لا نهاية له ولا بحسب أصنافها العامّية لأنّ المتباينة تباينا كثيرا لا يتصّل بعضها ببعض ولكن بحسب حركاتها.

[55] فنقول إنّ من الأمراض ما هي في غاية الحدّة والسرعة ومنها حادّة ومنها من سقوط {65B} الأمراض | الحادّة ووقوعها إلى المزمنة ومنها مزمنة طويلة المدّة والأمراض التي في غاية الحدّة منها ما هي في غاية القصوى من الحدّة بمنزلة الحمّى المطبقة التي تنقضي في أربعة

أيّام ومنها في الغاية٥ بمنزلة الحمّى المحرقة التي تقلع في سبعة أيّام وأمّا الأمراض الحادّة فمنها ما هي في الغاية من الحدّة وهي التي تنقضي في أربعة عشر يوما ومنها حادّة حدّة مرسلة وهي التي تنقضي في عشرين يوما. وأمّا الأمراض التي تكون من وقوع الحادّة الي المزمنة فمنها ما يكون دائمة ومنها ما يكون بنوائب وأمّا الأمراض المزمنة فمنها ما ينقضي في شهرين ومنها في سبعة أشهر ومنها في سبع سنين ومنها في أربعة عشر سنة.

[56] الأمراض منها حادّة وهي التي تكون مدّتها يسيرة ويكون صاحبها منها على خطر بمنزلة الحمّى المحرقة ومنها قصيرة المدّة وهي التي يقلّ مكثها ولا يكون معها خطر بمنزلة حمّى يوم ومنها ما يكون من وقوع الأمراض الحادّة إلى المزمنة وهي التي تكون حركتها في أوّل الأمر بطيئة ثمّ تحتدّ ومنها مزمنة وهي التي تكون حركتها منذ أوّل الأمر الى آخره حركة ليّنة.

[57] الأمراض منها ما هي في الغاية القصوى التي لا غاية بعدها من الحدّة وهي التي تنقضي في اليوم الرابع وينبغي أن يكون تدبير المريض في هذه أن يمسك عن الغذاء أصلا ومنها ما هي حادّة جدّا وليست في الغاية القصوى وهي التي تنقضي في اليوم السابع وينبغي أن يستعمل في هذه ماء العسل وحده ومنها ما هي خالصة الحدّة وهي التي تنقضي في أربعة عشر يوما وينبغي أن يستعمل فيها ماء كشك الشعير بحته كما هو ومنه ما يكون بوقوع الحادّة الى المزمنة ومنها مزمنة طويلة المدّة وهذه طبقات فمنها ما ينقضي في شهرين ومنها {66A} في سبعة أشهر ومنها في سبع سنين ومنها في أربعة عشرة سنة | وهذه ينبغي أن يكون التدبير فيها غليظا.

[58] الأمراض التي تنقضي في يوم الأربعين منها ما هي تلك التي تنقضي فيما بين أوّل المرض وبين تمام الأربعة عشر يوما ومنها ما يبتدئ أن يتحرّك حركات حادّة في الأيّام الباحورية التي بعد العشرين ومنها٦ ما يتهيأ فيه ذلك فيما بعد ويكون انقضاؤها إمّا في سبعة اشهر وإمّا في سبع سنين وإمّا في اربعة عشر سنة.

٥ الغاية: أيّ لا القصوى P1

٦ ومنها: أيّ من الأمراض التي هي مزمنة P1

[59] جالينوس يجعل حدود الأمراض الحادّة يوم الأربعة عشر ويوم الأربعين وحدود الأمراض التي من وقوع الأمراض الحادّة الى المزمنة يوم لأربعين ويوم الستّين.

[60] الأمراض التي يأتيها البحران في يوم العشرين هي إمّا الأمراض التي تبتدئ أن تتحرّك حركات بطيئة ثم أنّها من بعد اليوم الرابع أو السابع تتحرّك حركات حادّة وإمّا الأمراض التي يأتيها بحران على غير تمام.

[61] تمّت جوامع المقالة الثانية من كتاب جالينوس في أيّام البحران والحمد لله ربّ العالمين وصلواته على نبيّه محمّد وآله الطاهرين.

[62] {66B} | بسم الله الرحمن الرحيم الله ولي التوفيق

جوامع المقالة الثالثة من كتاب جالينوس في أيّام البحران

الأصول التي منها تستخرج معرفة أيّام البحران أصلين أحدهما يصحّ بما يشهد به التجربة والآخر بما يشهد به القياس.

[63] أشكال القمر سبعة أربعة منها تكون قبل الامتلاء[٧] وثلثة بعد الامتلاء أمّا الأربعة التي قبل الامتلاء فالواحد منها يقال له باليونانية مينوايدس وهو المستهلّ ويسمّى المسدّس [M4] والثاني يقال له باليونانية دمحوطوس وتفسيره (| في الهامش: الأسماء اليونانية لم أجدها في النصّ؟) المقسوم بنصفين ويسمّى المربّع والثالث يقال له باليونانية امفيقورطن وتفسيره ذو الحدّتين ويسمّى المثلّث والرابع يقال له باليونانية فانسالنين وهو الامتلاء والبدر وتسمّى القطر وأمّا الثلثة التي بعد الامتلاء فهي ذو الحدّتين والمقسوم بنفصين والمحاق.

[64] الشمس إذا صارت فوق رؤوسنا صار الزمان صيفا وإذا انحطّت وصارت إلى ناحية الجنوب صار الزمان شتاء وإذا صارت في الحمل صار الزمان ربيعا وإذا صارت في الميزان صار الزمان خريفا.

---

٧ الامتلاء: أي بقبل الامتلاء ومعه P¹

[65] الذي يحدث في الهواء من رؤية الهلال وإلى محاقه أنّ في وقت الاجتماع تتغيّر تغيّرات قوية جدّا طويلة المدّة جدّا وعند الامتلاء تتغيّر تغيّرات قوية إلّا أنّها تكون قليلة المكث وعند التنصيف تتغيّر تغيّرات عظيمة وعند التحدّب تتغيّر تغيّرات ضعيفة وعند المحاق تتغيّر تغيّرات لا بال بها.

[66] رؤية الهلال تسرع وتبطئ لأربعة أسباب وذلك أنّه مرّة يرى في اليوم الثاني ومرّة يرى في اليوم الثالث والسبب في ذلك إمّا من قبل حركته الخاصّية وإمّا من احتلاف العرض وإمّا من قبل وقت الاجتماع وإمّا من قبل احتلاف العرض.

[67] {67A} أسابيع دور القمر أربعة أحدها منذ وقت رؤيته | إلى أن ينقسم بنصفين وذلك يكون في الثور والأسد على تربيع والثاني إلى وقت ما يصير بدرا وذلك يكون في العقرب والدلو على تربيع والثالث إلى وقت ما يصير مقسوما بنصفين في النقصان وذلك يكون في الحمل والسرطان على تربيع والرابع إلى وقت الاستتار جملة وذلك يكون في الميزان والجدي على تربيع.

[68] أدوار أيّام البحران

الأدوار الباحورية منها أيّامية ومنها شهورية ومنها سنوية وأمّا الأيّامية فاليوم الرابع والسابع والرابع عشر وأمّا الشهورية فيوم الأربعين والستّة الأشهر وأمّا السنوية فالسبع سنين والأربعة عشر سنة. قياس الأدوار إلى أشباهها يجري على هذا منزلة الأربعة عشر إذا قيس بدور القمر فكان على قطر بمنزلة الستّة الأشهر إذا قيست بدور الشمس ومنزلة الأربعة عشر ‹سنة› إذا قيست بدور زحل. وأيضا منزلة اليوم السابع من دور القمر هي منزلة مدّة الثلثة الأشهر من دور الشمس ومنزلة السبع سنين من دور زحل وعلى هذا المثال أيضا فإنّ منزلة اليوم الرابع من دور القمر إذا كان على التسديس هي بمنزلة يوم الخمسة والأربعين من دور الشمس.

[69] مبدأ الأمراض يجري على وجهين أحدهما المبدأ الذي نراه عيانا في كون كلّ واحد منها والآخر المبدأ الذي يتغيّر في الهواء من قبل الشمس في كلّ شهر ومن قبل القمر في

كلّ أسبوع.

[70] الذي يضطرّ الأمراض إلى أن يتقدّم بحرانها هو شدّة المرض وصعوبته في نفسه والخطأ الذي يعترض إمّا من قبل الطبيب وإمّا من قبل المريض وإمّا ممّن يحضره من أهله وخاصّة خدمه وإمّا من الاشياء التى تعرض من خارج. أيّام البحران الواقعة في الوسط هي في الأمراض الحادّة كثيرة أعني الثالث والخامس والسادس والتاسع وفي الأمراض {67B} | المزمنة يسيرة.

[71] القوّة الدافعة التي في البدن ربّما تحرّكت إلى دفع الفضل قبل النضج التامّ بسبب شيء يزعجها ويحثّها على ذلك إمّا من خارج وإمّا من داخل. أمّا من خارج فمن الطبيب أو من المريض أو من أهله وخاصّته أو من الاشياء التي تعرض من خارج وأمّا من داخل فصعوبة المرض والخلط المؤذي ونوبة الحمّى وأسباب هذه كلّها ربّما تحرّكت إلى ذلك حركة بطيئة بعد استحكام النضج بسبب ضعفها.

[72] نوبة الحمّى تتحرّك في حمّى البلغم في كلّ يوم وفي حمّى الغبّ يوما ويوما لا وفي حمّى الربع يوما ويومين لا.

[73] أصحاب بوثاغورس يزعمون أنّ الأعداد صنفان فمنها أفراد وهي ذكورة بمنزلة الثالث والخامس والسابع والتاسع والثالث يأتي فيها البحران بسبب شدّة الدور واستكراهه والخامس بسبب قوّة الطبيعة والسابع بسبب القمر والتاسع بسبب الخطأ العارض إذا كان عظيما ومنها أزواج وهي إناث بمنزلة اليوم الثاني والرابع والسادس والثامن والعاشر.

[74] الأمراض منها ما تكون نوائبها متّصلة بمنزلة الحمّى المحرقة وهي التي تكون هيجانها وصعوبتها يوما ويوما لا ومنها ما هي من جنس الأمراض المزمنة إلّا أنّها تتحرّك حركات حادّة بمنزلة الحمّى المركّبة من حمّى البلغم وحمّى الغبّ ومنها ما تكون دائمة مطبقة بمنزلة حمّى الدم وهي التي تكون الحمّى فيها على مثال واحد في جميع الأيّام.

[75] اليوم العشرون هو من أيّام البحران لسببين أحدهما وهو الأوّل أنّ الأمراض التي تطول مدّتها ويكون هيجانها وصعوبتها في أيّام أزواج إنّما تنقضي في يوم من أيّام

الأزواج والثاني أنّ الأسبوع ليس هو سبعة أيّام تامّة وذلك أنّ السنة إنّما هي ثلثمائة وخمسة وستّون | {68A} يوما وربع يوم والشهر تسعة وعشرون يوما وسدس يوم والأسبوع ستّة أيّام ونصف وسدس.

[76] الأسابيع يضاف بعضها إلى بعض إضافات مختلفة فالأسبوع الثاني يوصل بالأسبوع الأوّل صلّة افتراق والثالث يوصل بالثاني صلّة اتّصال.

[77] الأرابيع أيضا يتّصل بعضها ببعض اتّصالات مختلفة فالرابوع الأوّل يوصل بالثاني صلّة اتّصال والثاني يوصل بالثالث صلّة افتراق والرابع يوصل بالثالث صلّة اتّصال والخامس يوصل بالرابع صلّة اتّصال والسادس يوصل بالخامس صلّة اتّصال.

[78] الأمراض طبقات فمنها حادّة وضدّها الأمراض المتريّثة البطيئة الحركة ومنها مزمنة طويلة المدّة وضدّها الأمراض القصيرة المدّة ومنها كثيرة المكث وضدّها حمّى يوم.

تمّت جوامع المقالة الثالثة من كتاب جالينوس في أيّام البحران وتمّ الكتاب بأسره والحمد لله ربّ العالمين وصلّى الله على نبيّه محمّد وآله الطاهرين.

2 Tehran MS

[1] بسم الله الرحمن الرحيم رب يسّر

أصناف البحران ستّة أحدها التغيّر السريع المائل إلى الصحّة، ويقال له بالحقيقة بحرانا جيّدا، ويتقدّمه إمّا استفراغ موثوق به وإمّا خراج عظيم. والاستفراغ يكون إمّا بالرعاف وإمّا بالعرق وإمّا باستطلاق البطن وإمّا بالبول وإمّا بالدم الذي يخرج من أفواه العروق التي هي المقعدة وإمّا بدرور الطمث. والخراج العظيم يكون إمّا في واحد من المفاصل وإمّا في واحد من الأعضاء التي لا شرف لها، والثاني التغيّر السريع المائل إلى الموت ويقال له بحرانا رديئا أعني الغشي، والثالث التغيّر الذي يؤول بصاحبه إلى الصحّة في مدّة من الزمان طويل ويقال له نضج المرض، والرابع التغيّر الذي يؤول بصاحبه إلى الموت في مدّة طويلة ويقال له الذبول، والخامس التغيّر المركّب من السريع والبطيء الذي يؤول بصاحبه إلى الصحّة والسلامة ويقال له بحرانا مركّبا جيّدا، والسادس التغيّر المركّب الذي يؤول بصاحبه إلى الموت ويقال له بحرانا مركّبا رديئا.

[2] الأيّام منها ما يأتي فيه البحران ومنها ما لا يأتي فيه بحران، والتي يأتي فيها البحران منها ما يكون فيه بحران جيّد تامّ. ويتمّ ذلك فيها مرارا كثيرة ويكون البحران فيها مأمون العاقبة وحريز من الآفات العارضة بعده وظاهرا. وقد تقدّم الإنذار به وجيّدا بمنزلة اليوم السابع.

[3] ومنها ما تجتمع فيه سبع خصال أضداد لتلك، وهو أن يكون البحران غير تامّ وأن يكون في الندرة وأن يشرف منه صاحبه[٨] على خطر عظيم ولا يؤمن عاقبته ولا يكون ظاهرا ولا يتقدّم الإنذار به ويكون رديئا بمنزلة اليوم السادس. وأمّا الأيّام التي لا يأتي فيها بحران فبمنزلة اليوم الثاني عشر والثالث عشر.

---

٨ صاحبه: منه add T

[4] الأمراض تعاود بنكسة يكون منها بعضها هي أمراض مهلكة قتّالة وهي التي تكون القوّة فيها قد خارت وضعفت وظهرت معها علامات العطب والتلف، وبعضها لا تكون قتّالة ولكن[٩] ينكس صاحبها. وماكان من الأمراض كذلك فهي من قبل أنّ القوّة تكون فيها صحيحة قوية لا تقتل لأنّ القوّة تكرّ على المرض ثانية فتجاهده حتّى تقهره.

[5] وبعضها يمكن فيه أن تمنع من العودة والنكسة وهي الأمراض السليمة التي ليس معها أعراض رديّة. فإنّ التدبير الملطّف يبلغ في هذه الأمراض ما يحتاج إليه من منع المرض من العودة والنكسة.

[6] ينبغي أن يستعمل في الأمراض التي يكون الإنسان منها على الثقة عند انقضائها التدبير المنعش حتّى يردّ المريض إلى تدبيره كان في وقت صحّته قليلا قليلا بركوب الخيل والجلوس على الفحل والأسرّة التي تحرّك وبدخول الحمّام وبشرب الشراب الموافق وأكل الطعام الملائم بمنزلة لحم الفراريج والسمك الرضراضي.

[7] وأمّا في الأمراض التي قد سكنت سكونا ليس صاحبه على ثقة منه فينبغي أن يكون التدبير مثل تدبير المرضى وذلك أنّه إن كان المرض الذي سكن مرضا يسير المقدار منعه هذا التدبير من أن يعاود لأنّ الأمراض الليّنة التي ليس معها أعراض خبيثة رديّة قد يمكن فيها أن تمنع من المعاودة. وإن كان المرض عظيم المقدار خبيثا ثمّ دبّرت المريض[١٠] بمثل التدبير الذي كان يتدبّر به في وقت مرضه كانت معاودة المرض له معاودة لا يشرف بها على الخطر، وإن دبّرته لا يحرز[١١] له فيه، كانت نكسته نكسة خطر.

[8] علامات البحران منها ما يكون بسبب العضو الدافع للفضل بمنزلة انجذاب مراقّ البطن إلى فوق، ومنها ما يكون بسبب العضو المؤدّي والمنفذ للفضل بمنزلة ضيق النفس. ومنها ما يكون بسبب العضو القابل للفضل بمنزلة الدموع والصداع واختلاط الذهن

٩ لكن: emendation eds ليكن T

١٠ المريض: emendation eds المرض T

١١ يحرز: emendation eds يجوز T

والسبات وثقل الصدغين ووجع الرقبة وخفقان الفؤاد والنافض. ومنها ما يكون بسبب الفضل نفسه بمنزلة اللمع الذي يراه الإنسان وإظلام البصر.

[9] وجود حقيقة أيّام البحران عسر شاقّ لأنّ مبدأ المرض يعسّر حركة إدراكه والوقوف عليه، ولأنّ البحران ربّما امتدّ أيّاما كثيرة ولأجل ذلك فمن الناس من يقول إنّ اليوم الأوّل هو يوم البحران أعني اليوم الذي فيه ابتداء البحران بأن يكون، ومنهم من يقول إنّ اليوم الأوّل والثاني هو يوم البحران وهو اليوم الذي فيه يظهر أكثر زمان البحران، ومنهم من يقول إنّ اليوم الثالث هو يوم البحران وهو اليوم الذي فيه يحلّ المرض. يوم البحران بالحقيقة هو اليوم الذي يجتمع فيه جميع أعلام البحران. وأقلّ منه في عدد أيّام البحران اليوم الذي تنقص فيه علامات البحران علامة أو علامتين. واليوم الذي يميل فيه المرض ميلا لا يستقيم فيه البحران هو اليوم الذي تكون فيه من علامات البحران وينقص منها ثلاثة.

[10] الأيّام الباحورية منها ما يكون فيه البحران أكثر وهي أيّام جياد بمنزلة اليوم السابع، فإنّ هذا اليوم يأتي فيه البحران في كثير من المرضى ويكون بحرانه جيّدا تامّا مأمون العاقبة سليما من الخطر قد تقدّم الإنذار به، وذلك أنّ اليوم الرابع ينذر به بتغيّر يحدث فيه بمنزلة النضج الذي يتبيّن إمّا في البول أو في النفث أو في البراز وإمّا في الفعل أعني الشهوة والحسّ والعقل والنوم.

[11] ومنها ما يكون فيه البحران أقلّ وهي أيّام رديّة بمنزلة اليوم السادس فإنّ هذا أيضا يأتي فيه البحران في قليل من المرضى ويكون بحرانه رديّا غير تامّ وغير ظاهر ولا مأمون العاقبة ولا سليم من الخطر.

[12] ومنها ما لا يكون فيه بحران بمنزلة اليوم الثاني عشر واليوم السادس عشر.

[13] قد اختلف الناس في التغيّر الحادث في المرض، فسمّى بعضهم كلّ تغيّر يحدث في المرض دفعة بحرانا، وبعضهم يسمّي بحرانا التغيّر الذي إلى السلامة وبعضهم يسمّي بحرانا ما يتقدّم من الاضطراب خاصّة إن يكون بحثهم عن الأمور أنفسها وخاصّة أصحاب

الجدل إن يبحثوا عن صحّة أسمائها وإجرائها مجاريها وخاصّة أصحاب اللغة وتقويمها والخطباء البحث عن الأسماء المألوفة والأسماء الغريبة .

[14] إذا كان من شأن التغيّر إلى الحال الأردى أن يحدث في اليوم السادس فإنّه يتقدّم ذلك في اليوم الرابع صغر نفس وبرد ورعدة وخور وعرق غير مستو في البدن واستفراغ أشياء لم تنضج .

[15] الأيّام الباحورية منها ما لا يزال البحران يأتي فيها دائما ومنها ما لا يكاد فيه يأتي البحران إلاّ في الندرة ومنها ما حالها في ذلك حال وسط . فأمّا الأيّام التي يكون فيها البحران دائما فمنها ما هي في الطبقة الأولى من طبقات أيّام البحران بمنزلة اليوم السابع والعاشر واليوم الرابع عشر، ومنها في الطبقة الثانية بمنزلة اليوم التاسع والتاسع عشر والعشرين، ومنها في الطبقة الثالثة بمنزلة اليوم السابع عشر واليوم الخامس، ومنها في الطبقة الرابعة بمنزلة اليوم الرابع والثالث والثامن عشر .

[16] وأمّا الأيّام التي لا يكاد البحران يأتي فيها إلّا في الندرة، وذلك في ثلاث طبقات، منها ما هو في الطبقة الأولى بمنزلة اليوم الخامس والسادس ومنها في الطبقة الثانية بمنزلة اليوم الثامن واليوم الخامس عشر ومنها في الطبقة الثالثة بمنزلة اليوم الثاني عشر .

وأمّا الأيّام التي حالها حال وسط بين هذه فهي بمنزلة اليوم الثالث عشر واليوم السادس عشر .

[17] مبدأ المرض عند بعض الناس هو وقت الإحساس بالأذى وعند بعضهم هو مبدأ إلقاء الإنسان نفسه، والناس في هذا الإلقاء مختلفون فمنهم من يلقي نفسه قبل أن يكون المرض لخوره وضعف نفسه. ومنهم من يفعل ذلك بعد حدوث المرض لقوّة نفسه وشدّة صبره واحتماله، ومنهم من يمنعه اشتغاله بأمر دنياه من أن يلقي نفسه فلا يلقيها إلّا في آخر الأمر . وعند بعض الناس مبدأ المرض هو الوقت الذي يحسّ فيه العليل بمبدأ أضرار المرض به .

[18] المرضى منهم من يعرض له المرض دفعة من غير أن يتقدّم ذلك علامات تدلّ عليه،

ومنهم من لا يعرض له المرض دفعة لكن بعد ما ينالهم الأذى وتحدث بهم أعراض المرض، فيكون أوّل ما يعرض لهم الأذى ثمّ تبتدئ بآخره بهم الحمّى.

[19] مبدأ المرض على ضربين إمّا بحسب الطبيعة، وهو المبدأ الذي نقول فيه إنّه يتبيّن بالقياس، وإمّا بحسب الحسّ وهو المعروف، وعليه ينبغي أن تعمل [?] الدلائل التي على طريق المثال إمّا ما يدلّ منها على البحران. فاليوم الذي قد سبق فأنذر بدلالة جيّدة. فأمّا الدالّة على ظهوره فالأعراض الباحورية والقشعريرية والعرق. فأمّا التي لا تدلّ على خطر فهي الغريبة من الأعراض، فأمّا كماله فالخلاص من الحمّى وأمّا التي على حدوثه فالبلوغ إلى الخلاص. فأمّا الدالّة على الثقة فجميع هذه معا.

[20] متى كان البحران في يومين ولم يكن يتقدّمه يوم ينذر به، فينبغي أن تستخرج معرفة اليوم الذي هو يوم البحران من قياس الأدوار من طبيعة اليوم ومن عدد الأيّام الباحورية ومن وقت البحران.

[21] الأوقات التي تكون فيها البحران ثلاثة، أحدها وقت النوبة والثاني وقت الاستفراغ والثالث وقت التخلّص من المرض. وهذه الثلاثة الأوقات إن حضرت في يوم واحد قلنا إنّ ذلك اليوم يوم بحران، فإن كانت في يومين فليس ينبغي أن يسمّى يوم البحران إلّا اليوم الذي أنذر به اليوم المنذر إذا كان البحران في يومين. إن وجدت أكثر الأعراض الباحورية في اليوم الأوّل منهما ووجد شيئا منها أيضا في اليوم الثاني فينبغي أن يعطى اليوم الثاني جزء من البحران، فإن وجدت تلك الأعراض في اليومين عامّة فالبحران هو عامّ لهما جميعا.

[22] أيّام البحران التي بعد يوم العشرين عند أصحاب بقراط وجالينوس في يوم العشرين والرابع والعشرين والسابع والعشرين والواحد والثلاثين والرابع والثلاثين والسابع والثلاثين والأربعين. وهي عند أصحاب أرجنجانس اليوم الواحد والعشرين والثامن والعشرين والثاني والأربعين والخامس والأربعين والثامن والأربعين.

[23] الأدوار المتناسبة هي ثلاثة أعني دور القمر ودور الشمس ودور زحل، وقد ذكر

بقراط يوم الأربعين ويوم الستّين ويوم الثمانين و يوم المائة والعشرين.

[24] الخروج من المرض يكون مع جهاد قويّ شديد إلى اليوم الرابع عشر ومع جهاد معتدل قصد إلى اليوم الأربعين ولا يكون معه الجهاد إلّا في الندرة فيما بين الأربعين من الأمراض التي انقضاؤها يكون على جهة المجاورة وهي التي يمتدّ فيها البحران إلى ثلاثة أيّام.

[25] ‹قال جالينوس› إنّه ينبغي لمن أراد أن يتقدّم فيعرف يوم البحران أن يكون عالما بتقدمة المعرفة التي أفادها بقراط وأن يكون قد جرّب واحتنك في مزاولة المرضى بالفعل وأن يكون متقنا لعلم النبض

[26] العلامات منها ما يدلّ على النجاة ومنها على العطب ومنها على الخطر ومنها على نضج المرض.

[27] فالعلامات الدالّة على السلامة هي أن تكون القوّة قوية والتنفّس سهلا والمريض خفيف البدن وأن يكون النبض حسنا.

[28] والعلامات الدالّة على العطب هي سوء التنفّس وثقل البدن ورداءة النبض. فأمّا علامات الخطر فالعرق البارد وأمّا علامات النضج فالبول النضيج.

[29] الخطأ العارض من جهة المريض إن كان يسير المقدار حدث بسببه في اليوم السابع بحران غير تامّ، وإن كان عظيم المقدار حدث عنه ذلك إمّا في اليوم التاسع أو في اليوم الحادي عشر. وإذا كان الخطأ من جهة المريض، أمّا في الأمراض التي لا خطر فيها فإنّها تتطاول ويزمن تحلّلها، وأمّا في الأمراض التي فيها خطر فإنّها تؤول إلى التلف، وأمّا التي تفضي إلى الخلاص فإنّها تكون خطرا. الخطأ يكون إمّا من قبل الطبيب وإمّا من قبل المريض وإمّا من قبل خدمه وإمّا من قبل الأشياء التي ترد من خارج بمنزلة الصياح وخصومة الجيران وسماع الحرب وورود خبر يغمّ. البحران في الأمراض التي تؤول إلى السلامة يتأخّر، وفي الأمراض القتّالة يتقدّم كونه. فأمّا الأمراض التي لا خطر فيها ويتأخّر البحران فيها فإنّه إن كان ذلك في اليوم الخامس فإنّ المرض يكون حادّا ونوائبه في أيّام أفراد والخطر يكون عظيما. فإن كان في اليوم السادس فإنّ الأحوال تكون بالضدّ.

[30] من الأمراض ما يمكننا أن نتعرّف منذ أوّل الأمر نوع كلّ واحد منها وآخر ما ينتهي إليه بمنزلة الحمّى الغبّ. إذا كانت حمّى تبين ولم يتبيّن فيها في الأيّام الأول علامات النضج ومنها ما يعرف نوعها ولا يعرف آخر ما ينتهي إليه بمنزلة الحمّى البلغم المتطاولة.

[31] الأمراض منها ما هو سليم، وانقضاؤها يكون في اليوم الرابع وعلامات النضج تتبيّن فيها منذ أوّل يوم. وما كان كذلك فينبغي أن يدبّر صاحبه بألطف التدبير وأدقّه، ومنها ما هو قتّال وانقضاؤه يكون في اليوم الرابع ومنها ما هو سليم إلّا أنّ معه علامات تدلّ على أنّ المرض لم ينضج وربّما كانت معه علامات تدلّ على أنّه سيطول. فإن اجتمعت فيها هاتان الخصلتان فهو مرض يطول وينبغي أن يدبّر صاحبه تدبيرا غليظا. وإن كانت فيه واحدة من الخصلتين أعني علامة تدلّ على أنّ المرض لم ينضج فقط فهو مرض يكون أقلّ طولا وينبغي أن يدبّر صاحبه تدبيرا أقلّ غلظا.

[32] علامات النضج إن تبيّنت في اليوم الرابع فإنّ البحران يكون في اليوم السابع وإن تبيّنت في اليوم السابع فالبحران يأتي في اليوم الرابع عشر، وإن تبيّنت في الرابع عشر فالبحران يأتي إمّا في اليوم السابع عشر وإمّا في الثامن عشر وإمّا في العشرين وإمّا في الواحد والعشرين. فإنّ اليوم السابع عشر هو منذر بأحد هذين اليومين

[33] إذا كان المرض يطول وتبيّنت فيه علامات تدلّ على أنّه لم ينضج أو على أنّه يطول فإنّ تلك العلامات إن تبيّنت إلى اليوم السابع دلّت على أنّ المرض لا ينقضي في اليوم الرابع عشر، وإن تبيّنت إلى اليوم الحادي عشر فالمرض ينقضي من بعد اليوم العشرين، وإن تبيّنت إلى اليوم السابع عشر فالمرض ينقضي في اليوم الأربعين.

[34] تمّت جوامع الاسكندرانيين للمقالة الأولى من كتاب جالينوس في أيّام البحران والحمد لله وحده كثيرا

[35] بسم الله الرحمن الرحيم

الأسباب في اختلاف آراء الناس في أمر أيّام البحران ثلاثة، أحدها أنّ الوقوف على مبدأ المرض عسر شاقّ، والثاني للخطأ العارض إمّا من قبل الطبيب وإمّا من قبل المريض

وإمّا من قبل خدمه وإمّا من الأشياء التي تعرض من خارج، والثالث أنّ البحران ربّما امتدّ أيّاما كثيرة.

[36] الأيّام منها أيّام بحران ومنها أيّام إنذار ومنها أيّام واقعة في الوسط. فأمّا أيّام البحران فالرابع والسابع والحادي عشر والرابع عشر والسابع عشر والعشرين، وأمّا الأيّام التي تنذر بأيّام البحران فالرابع والحادي عشر والرابع عشر، فأمّا الأيّام الواقعة في الوسط فالثالث والخامس والسادس والثالث عشر والخامس عشر.

[37] أرابيع أيّام البحران يختلف عددها. فالرابوع الأوّل والرّابوع الثاني يعدّان متّصلين والرابوع الثاني مع الرابوع الثالث يعدّان مفترقين والرابوع الثالث مع الرابع يعدّان متّصلين والرابع والخامس أيضا يعدّان معا متّصلين لأنّ الخامس ينتهي في اليوم السابع عشر. وعلى هذا المثال أيضا فالخامس والسادس يعدّان معا ومتّصلين.

[38] جميع القدماء قد اتّفقوا على أنّ أيّام البحران إلى اليوم الرابع عشر. فأمّا في الأيّام التي من بعد هذا اليوم فقد اختلفوا وذلك أنّ قوما منهم يزعمون إلى أيّام البحران التي من بعد اليوم الرابع عشر هي اليوم السابع عشر واليوم العشرين واليوم الواحد والعشرين واليوم السابع والعشرين واليوم الواحد والثلاثين واليوم الرابع والثلاثين واليوم الأربعين واليوم الثمانين واليوم المائة والعشرين. وقوم آخرون يزعمون أنّ أيّام البحران التي من بعد اليوم الرابع عشر هي اليوم الثامن عشر واليوم الواحد والعشرين واليوم الخامس والعشرين واليوم الثامن والعشرين واليوم الثاني والثلاثين واليوم الخامس والثلاثين واليوم الثاني والأربعين واليوم الرابع والثمانين.

[39] كتاب بقراط المسمّى أبيديميا سبع مقالات، منها صحيحة لا شكّ وهي الأولى والثالثة ومنها مشكوك في أمرها وهي الثانية والرابعة والسادسة ومنها منحولة وهي الخامسة والسابعة.

[40] إذا كانت الأمراض ممّا تتطاول مدّة البحارين فيها فينبغي أن تتعرّف يوم البحران من مبادئ الأمراض ومن الأيّام المنذرة بالبحران ومن حركات نوائب المرض.

[41] البحارين منها ما تكون محدودة وهي التي تبدأ وتنقض‹ي› في يوم واحد. ومنها غير محدودة وهي التي تتمادى أيّاما كثيرة.

[42] الراحة من الأمراض تكون على ثلاثة أنحاء إمّا بالنضج عندما يفنى الخلط الذي هو بسبب المرض أو بالاستفراغ إذا اندفع السبب الفاعل للمرض بأسره إلى خارج أو ‹ب›خراج أو ‹ب›قرحة إذا اندفع ذلك الشيء إلى الأعضاء غير الشريفة.

[43] الأمراض المزمنة منها ما يحلّ بطريق النضج ومنها ما يكون انحلالها أخيرا دفعة بحركة سريعة[١٢]. وأيضا فمن الأمراض المزمنة ما يتمادى البحران فيها أيّاما كثيرة. ومنها ما يبتدئ وينقضي بحرانه في يوم واحد.

[44] طبيعة أيّام البحران مضاعفة وذلك أنّ منها ما هي بالطبع باحورية بمنزلة الرابع والسابع والرابع عشر والعشرين. ومنها ما يظنّ باحورية بمنزلة الثالث والخامس والتاسع والثالث عشر.

[45] المنفعة في العلم بأمر البحران مضاعفة وذلك أنّ منها ما ينتفع به في تقدمة معرفة البحارين، فإنّا قد نقف من الأشياء المنذرة بهذه على أنّها توجد. والمنفعة الثانية هي الوقوف على تحديد رسم التدبير. فإنّا إذا تقدّمت عندنا المعرفة باليوم الذي فيه يكون انحلال المرض كان رسمنا وتقديرنا التدبير بحسب ذلك.

[46] إنّ بقراط قد ذكر الأيّام الباحورية بالطبع في كتاب الفصول وفي كتاب تقدمة المعرفة. فأمّا في المقالة الأولى من كتاب الفصول فلم يتكلّم في الأيّام الباحورية فقط بل وفي الأيّام المتوسّطة بينها.

[47] وهذه الأيّام، فمنها أزواج وهي السادس والثامن والعاشر والعشرين، ومنها ما هي أفراد وهي الثالث والخامس والتاسع.

[48] أدوار أيّام البحران منها ما تكون رباعية وهي إلى اليوم العشرين، ومنها سابوعية وهي

---

١٢ سريعة: emendation eds سريعا T

التي تكون من اليوم العشرين إلى الرابع والثلاثين، ومنها عشرية وهي الكائنة من اليوم الأربعين إلى اليوم الستّين.

[49] أسباب الاختلاف في أيّام البحران كثيرة، أحدها الجهل بالمعرفة بأيّام البحران التي هي بالطبع كذلك والمظنونة، والثاني اقتصار الطالب لها على طلبها بالكلام والقياس دون التجربة، والثالث أن يكون الإنسان متى رأى يوما من الأيّام قد وقع فيه بحران دفعة واحدة قضا عليه بأنه من أيّام البحران ولم ينتظر حتّى ينظر هل يكون فيه أيضا بحران مرارا آخر أم لا، والرابع أن لا يقف الإنسان على فصول أيّام البحران وجهات البحارين. الفصول قد تكون في الأمراض في أنحاء البحارين وفي أيّام البحران.

[50] أمّا التي تكون في الأمراض، فإنّها قد تحدث في مثل هذا الزمان حمّيات محرقة وفي زمان آخر حمّيات غبّ وفي آخر حمّى ربع. وأمّا التي في أنحاء البحارين، فإنّ منها ما يعرض فيها في هذا الزمان مثلا بفجر الدم، ومنها ما يكون بالعرق ومنها ما يكون بالقيء، وأمّا التي تكون في أيّام البحران فمنها ما يكون وجود البحران في هذا الوقت في السابع ومنها ما يكون ذلك فيه في اليوم العاشر بحسب الوقت ومنها ما يوجب الوقت أن يكون في الحادي عشر.

[51] الأيّام منها ما يكون باحورية فقط وهو اليوم السابع والرابع عشر والعشرين، ومنها ما هي باحورية ومنذرة بمنزلة الرابع والحادي عشر والسابع عشر، ومنها واقعة في أوساط هذه بمنزلة الثالث والخامس والتاسع والثالث عشر.

[52] مقايسة الأيّام تجري على هذا النحو. أمّا الأيّام التي قبل يوم العشرين، فالأسبوعان الأوّلان يعدّان على انفرادهما غير متّصلين، وأمّا الأسبوع الثالث فيعدّ مع اتّصال ومزاوجة الثاني، فأمّا الأيّام التي بعد العشرين فإنّ الأسبوعين الأولّين إذا عدّا على انفرادهما أوجبا بحران الرابع والثلاثين. والأسبوع الثالث إذا عدّ مع الأسبوع الثاني من هذين كان عدّه اليوم الأربعين.

[53] الأدوار ثلاثة أحدها دور النصف الجانب عن مضاعفة الروابيع لأنّ الأربعة إذا ضوعفت حدث عنها الثمانية والإثنى عشر والستّة عشر. والثاني دور تامّ وهو الكائن عن

مضاعفة السوابيع بمنزلة الرابع عشر والحادي والعشرين[١٣] والثامن والعشرين والخامس والثلاثين والثاني والأربعين. والثالث وهو الأتمّ والأكمل وهو دور العشرين، فإنّ عن مضاعفته تحدث الأربعون والستّون والثمانون والمائة والعشرون.

[54] ينبغي أن تجعل قسمة الأمراض لا بحسب الأيّام الباحورية لأنّها غير محدودة ولا أيضا بفصولها الجنسية لأنّ بعضها لا يتّصل ببعض إذا كان تباينها شديدا بل يجب أن تكون قسمتها بحسب حركاتها.

[55] بأن نقول إنّ من الأمراض ما هي حادّة جدّا وهي تنقسم قسمين أحدهما في الغاية القصوى من الحدّة بمنزلة الحمّى المطبقة التي تسمّى سونوحس التي يكون انحلالها في اليوم الرابع. والقسم الآخر وهي الحادّة جدّا على الإطلاق بمنزلة الحمّى المحرقة التي انحلالها يكون في اليوم السابع، ومنها ما هي حادّة وهي تنقسم أيضا قسمين وذلك أنّ منها ما تكون حادّة بآخره وهي الأمراض التي يكون انحلالها على الإطلاق إلى اليوم الرابع عشر، ومنها ما هي حادّة على الإطلاق وهي الأمراض التي انحلالها يكون إلى اليوم العشرين. ومن الأمراض ما يحدث عن انحطاط الأمراض الحادّة وهي تنقسم قسمين وذلك أنّ منها ما تكون دائمة ومنها ما تكون نائبة. ومن الأمراض ما تكون مزمنة وأقسامها أربعة وذلك أنّ منها ما يكون انحلاله[١٤] في شهرين ومنها ما كون انحلاله في سبعة أشهر ومنها ما يكون انحلاله في سبع سنين ومنها ما يكون انحلاله في أربع عشرة سنة.

[56] الأمراض منها حادّة، وهي التي تكون مدّتها قصيرة والخطر فيها عظيما بمنزلة الحمّى المحرقة التي تسمّى قاوسوس. ومنها قصيرة المدّة يسيرة[١٥] الخطر بمنزلة حمّى يوم. ومنها ما يحدث عن انحطاط الأمراض الحادّة وهي التي تكون في أوّل أمرها بطيئة الحركة ثمّ تكون بآخره حادّة. ومنها ما هي مزمنة وهي التي تكون حركتها من الابتداء إلى الانتهاء

١٣ الحادي والعشرين: emendation eds الحادي عشر T

١٤ انحلاله: emendation eds بحرانه T

١٥ يسيرة: emendation eds يسير T

حركة بطيئة.

[57] الأمراض منها ما هي في غاية القصوى من الحدّة وهي التي يكون انحلالها في اليوم الرابع، وينبغي لنا في هذه الأمراض أن نمنع من الغذاء بالواحدة. ومنها حادّة جدّا على الإطلاق وهي التي تحلّ في اليوم السابع، ويجب أن يستعمل في هذه شراب العسل. ومنها ما هي حادّة على الحقيقة وهي التي يكون انحلالها في اليوم الرابع عشر، وينبغي أن يستعمل في هذه ماء الشعير. ومنها ما هي حادّة على الإطلاق وهي التي انحلالها يكون في اليوم العشرين، وفي هذه ينبغي أن يستعمل ماء الشعير بحتة[١٦] ومنها ما تكون حادّة حادثة عن انحطاط الأمراض، ومنها ما هي مزمنة وأقسامها أربعة وذلك أنّ منها ما يحلّ في شهرين ومنها ما يحلّ في سبعة أشهر ومنها ما يحلّ في سبع سنين ومنها في أربعة عشرة سنة، وينبغي أن يغلّظ التدبير في أمثال هذه الأمراض.

[58] الأمراض التي تحلّ في يوم الأربعين منها ما يحلّ قبل اليوم الرابع عشر ومنها ما يبتدأ باحتداد الحركة في الأيّام الباحورية من بعد اليوم العشرين ومنها ما يوجد لها ذلك فيما بعد ويكون انقضاؤها إمّا في سبعة أشهر وإمّا في سبع سنين وإمّا في أربع عشرة سنة.

[59] جالينوس يجعل أزمان الأمراض الحادّة إثنين، أحدها اليوم الرابع عشر والآخر اليوم الأربعين. فأمّا الأمراض الكائنة عن انحطاط أمراض أخر فإنّه يجعل لذلك أيضا زمانين أحدهما يوم الأربعين والآخر يوم الستّين.

[60] الأمراض التي يأتيها البحران في اليوم العشرين هي إمّا الأمراض التي تبطؤ حركتها في الابتداء ثمّ إنّها تبدأ[١٧] باحتداد الحركة بعد اليوم الرابع أو السابع أو تكون من الأمراض التي بحارينها غير تامّة.

[61] تمّت جوامع الاسكندرانيين للمقالة الثانية من كتاب جالينوس في أيّام البحران ولله الحمد والمنّة

١٦ بحتة: emendation eds بحره T

١٧ تبدأ: emendation eds يبداء T

[62] بسم الله الرحمن الرحيم
الأصول التي منها تستخرج معرفة أيّام البحران أصلان، أحدهما يصحّ بما تشهد به التجربة والثاني الذي يصحّ بطريق القياس.

[63] أشكال القمر سبعة، أربعة منها قبل الامتلاء وثلاثة بعد الامتلاء، أمّا الأربعة التي قبل الامتلاء فالواحد منها يقال له باليونانية مينوانداس وهو الهلالي ويسمّى ذو الستّ الزوايا والثاني يسمّى باليونانية دمخوطومون ومعناه المنصف ويسمّى ذو الأربع الزوايا، والثالث يقال له أمقيفورطون وتفسيره[18] ذو الحدبتين ويسمّى ذو الثلاث الزوايا، والرابع يقال له باليونانية فانسالينون وهو الامتلاء والبدر ويسمّى القطر. وأمّا الثلاثة التي بعد الامتلاء فهي ذو الحدبتين والمنصف والمحاق.

[64] الشمس إذا سامتت رؤوسنا كان الزمان صيفا. وإذا كانت منحطّة إلى ناحية الجنوب كان الزمان شتاء. وإذا كانت في الحمل كان الزمان ربيعا. وإذا كانت في الميزان كان الزمان خريفا.

[65] | الذي وقفنا عليه بالمشاهدة أنّ التغايير الحادثة عن الاجتماعات تكون قوية بطيئة جدّا. وعند الامتلاء تحدث تغايير قوية إلّا أنّها تكون قليلة المكث. وعند التنصّف تحدث تغايير عظيمة وعند التحدّب تحدث تغايير ضعيفة وعند المحاق تحدث تغايير ضعيفة. [66] | رؤية القمر تسرع وتبطئ لأربعة أسباب، وذلك أنّه مرّة يرى في اليوم الثاني ومرّة يرى في اليوم الثالث، والسبب في ذلك إمّا من قبل حركته الخاصّية وإمّا من قبل اختلاف العرض وإمّا من قبل وقت الاجتماع وإمّا من قبل الحركة المختلفة التي للبروج.

[67] أسابيع دور القمر أربعة أحدها منذ وقت رؤيته إلى أن ينتصف بنصفين وذلك يكون في الثور والأسد على تربيع، والثاني إلى وقت ما يصير بدرا. وذلك يكون في العقرب والدلو على تربيع، والثالث إلى ما يصير مقسوما بنصفين في النقصان وذلك يكون في الحمل

---

١٨ وتفسيره: emendation eds وتفسير T

والسرطان على تربيع، والرابع إلى وقت الاستتار بالجملة وذلك يكون في الميزان والجدي على تربيع.

[68] أدوار أيّام البحران منها يومية ومنها شهورية ومنها سنوية. أمّا اليومية فاليوم الرابع والسابع والرابع عشر. وأمّا الشهورية فيوم الأربعين والستّة الأشهر. وأمّا السنوية فالسبع سنين والأربع عشرة سنة.

قياس الأدوار على أسمائها يجري على هذا النحو، فنسبة الأربعة عشر يوما عند دور القمر هو القطر[١٩]، هي النسبة التي للستّة الأشهر عند دور الشمس، وهي النسبة التي للأربع عشرة سنة عند دور زحل وأيضا فإنّ النسبة الموجودة لليوم السابع عند الدور القمري والسبع سنين عند دور زحل هي بعينها النسبة للثلاثة الأشهر عند دور الشمس. وعلى هذا المثال أيضا فإنّ نسبة اليوم الرابع إلى دور القمر المسمّى ذو الستّ الزوايا هي النسبة الموجودة لليوم الخامس والأربعين عند دور الشمس.

[69] مبدأ الأمراض يجري على وجهين؛ أحدهما المبدأ الذي نراه عيانا في كون كلّ واحد منهما. والآخر المبدأ الذي يتغيّر فيه الهواء من قبل الشمس في كلّ شهر من قبل[٢٠] القمر في كلّ أسبوع.

[70] قد يجب ضرورة ويمكن أن يتقدّم بحارين الأمراض لسببين أحدهما قوّة النوبة والآخر لخطأ يعرض إمّا من قبل الطبيب أو من قبل المريض أو من قبل أهله وخدمه أو من قبل الأشياء التي من خارج. أيّام البحران الواقعة في الوسط هي في الأمراض الحادّة كثيرة أعني اليوم الثالث والخامس والسادس والتاسع، وفي الأمراض المزمنة يسيرة، الدور الأوّل إمّا في الأفراد فهو الثالث وإمّا في الأزواج فهو الرابع.

[71] القوّة الدافعة التي في البدن ربّما تحرّكت إلى دفع الفضل قبل النضج التامّ بسبب شيء يزعجها ويحثّها على ذلك إمّا من خارج وإمّا من داخل. أمّا من خارج فمن الطبيب أو من

---

١٩ القطر : emendation eds القطن T

٢٠ قبل: الأسبوع add T

المريض أو من أهله وخدمه أو من الأشياء التي تعرض من خارج، وأمّا التي من داخل فهي صعوبة المرض والخلط المؤذي والنوبة وأسباب هذه كلّها. وربّما تحرّكت إلى ذلك حركة بطيئة بعد استحكام النضج بسبب ضعفها.

[72] نوبة الحمّى تتحرّك في حمّى البلغم في كلّ يوم وفي الحمّى الغبّ في كلّ ثلاثة أيّام والحمّى الربع كلّ أربعة أيّام.

[73] أصحاب فوثاغورس يزعمون أنّ الأعداد تنقسم قسمين فمنها أفراد وهي ذكور ومنها أزواج وهي إناث، فأمّا الأفراد فهي الثالث والخامس والسابع والتاسع والحادي عشر. فالثالث يأتي فيه البحران بسبب قوّة الدور واستكراهه والخامس يأتي فيه البحران بسبب تعب الطبيعة والسابع يأتي فيه البحران بسبب القمر والتاسع بسبب الشمس والحادي عشر بسبب زحل، وأمّا الأزواج وهي الإناث فبمنزلة اليوم الثاني والرابع والسادس والثامن والعاشر.

[74] الأمراض منها ما تكون نوائبها متّصلة بمنزلة الحمّى المحرقة التي تسمّى قاوسوس وهي التي يكون هيجانها وصعوبتها كلّ ثلاثة أيّام ومنها ما هي من جنس الأمراض المزمنة إلّا أنّها تتحرّك حركات حادّة بمنزلة الحمّى المركّبة من حمّى البلغم وحمّى الغبّ، ومنها ما تكون دائمة مطبقة بمنزلة حمّى الدم وهي التي تكون الحمّى فيها على وتيرة واحدة في الأيّام كلّها.

[75] اليوم العشرين هو من أيّام البحران لشيئين، أحدهما وهو الأوّل أنّ الأمراض التي تطول مدّتها ويكون هيجانها وصعوبتها في أيّام الأزواج؛ فانحلالها يكون في يوم من أيّام الأزواج والثاني أنّ الأسبوع ليس هو سبعة أيّام تامّة وذلك أنّ السنة إنّما هي ثلثمائة وخمسة وستّين يوما وربع يوم والشهر تسعة وعشرين يوما وسدس والأسبوع ستّة أيّام وسدس.

[76] الأسابيع يضاف بعضها إلى بعض إضافات مختلفة، فالأسبوع الثاني يوصل بالأسبوع الأوّل صلة افتراق والثالث يوصل بالثاني صلة اتّصال.

[77] الروابيع أيضا تتّصل بعضها ببعض اتّصالا مختلفا. فالرابوع الأوّل يوصل بالثاني صلة اتّصال والثاني يوصل بالثالث صلة افتراق والرابع يوصل بالثالث صلة اتّصال والخامس

يوصل بالرابع صلة اتّصال والسادس يوصل بالخامس صلة اتّصال.

[78] الأمراض طبقات فمنها حادّة وضدّها المزمنة البطيئة الحركة ومنها طويلة المدّة وضدّها الأمراض القصيرة المدّة ومنها طويلة المكث وضدّها حمّى يوم.

تمّت جوامع الاسكندرانيين للمقالة الثالثة من كتاب جالينوس في أيّام البحران، وهي تمام الكتاب ولله الحمد والمنّة.

CHAPTER 4

The Translation of the Arabic Text

In the name of God, the Compassionate, the Merciful.
The summaries of the first book of Galen's book *On Critical Days*.

[1] There are six types of crisis. One is a swift change that tends towards health; it is truly called a good crisis.[1] It comes about by means of a trustworthy evacuation, or a severe inflammation. The evacuation will be either by sweat, by nosebleed, a bowel movement, urine, the blood that comes out from the mouths of the arteries in the buttocks, or by the menstrual flow.[2] The severe inflammation will be in one of the joints, or in one of the limbs that are not noble. The second is a swift change that tends towards death; it is called a bad, difficult crisis. The third is the change that eventually results in health for the one who experiences it, after a long period of time. It is called the ripening of the illness. The fourth is the change that eventually results in death for the patient, after a long period; it is called wasting. The fifth is the change that is compounded of the swift and the slow, and which results in health and safety for the patient. It is called a good compound crisis. The sixth is the compound crisis that results in death for the one who experiences it. It is called a bad compound crisis.

[2] The crisis comes on some days, and on others the crisis does not come. On some of the days on which the crisis comes, the crisis is good and complete. It has been disposed to do this[3] many times on them; the crisis on

---

1 The distinction between six types and their definitions does not feature in Galen. Galen merely states in the beginning of *On Critical Days* (K 769.1-4; CG 96-97), that "in order for the resolution of illnesses that do not diminish gradually, but that subsided all at once to be trustworthy, there must occur beforehand either an obvious bodily evacuation, or an evident inflammation." However, a similar distinction into six types recurs in the anonymous *Aggregationes de crisi et creticis diebus* (*The Summary on Crises and Critical Days*) that was composed in the thirteenth century. See C. Boyle (ed.), *Medieval Prognosis and Astrology: A Working Edition of the Aggregationes de crisi et creticis diebus: with Introduction and English Summary* (Cambridge 1991), p. 32. For this work see as well: F. Wallis (ed.), *Medieval Medicine. A Reader* (Toronto 2010), section 65: Panacea or Problem? (I): The case for medical astrology, pp. 318-323.

2 The symptoms mentioned here recur with some variations in K 770.6-13 (CG 96-98); thus for "sweat" Galen speaks of "a praiseworthy sweat over the whole body", and for "urine" he mentions "plentiful urine"; and for "severe inflammation will be in one of the joints" Galen has "an inflammation in the soft flesh below the ear".

3 *tahayyaʾa fīhā*, literally "it has become a disposition within it." MS Tehran reads here *yat-*

 | DOI 10.1163/9789004282223_005

them is sure of the outcome, protected against harmful things afterwards, and evident. There was an indication that it will be good, as is the case on the seventh day.[4]

[3] For others, seven characteristics that are the opposite of these come together, namely when the crisis is not complete. The patient is on the brink of great danger; its outcome is not sure and it is not clear. There was no indication for it, and it is bad as is the case on the sixth day.[5] As for the days on which the crisis [never][6] comes, [they are] the twelfth day and the sixteenth day.[7]

[4] Some of the illnesses which return with a relapse are destructive and fatal. Those are the ones in which the capacity [for healing] has dwindled and weakened; along with it, signs of ruin and destruction have appeared. Others are not fatal; instead, the one suffering from it has only had a relapse. When diseases are like this, it is because the faculty therein (in the body) is sound and strong. It is not fatal because the [healing] capacity attacks the illness a second time, exerting itself until it overcomes it.[8]

[5] In yet others it is able to prevent a return and relapse. These are the safe diseases that are not accompanied by bad symptoms. A thin regimen suffices here for what is necessary to prevent the disease from returning and relapsing.

[6] When diseases with regard to which the person is confident [of full recovery] terminate, the revitalizing regimen must be employed. It is the regimen for convalescents, such that the patient may return to the regimen

---

immu, "it will be completed", which makes no sense here.

4 The text in this section seems to be based on two statements found in Galen, at K 779.13-15 (CG 114-115) and K 775.10-12 (CG 106-107). Cf. *Aggregationes*, ed. Boyle, pp. 57-58, which mentions seven conditions for a day to be truly critical, and concludes that the virtue of a crisis is strongest in seven-day periods.

5 Cf. Galen, K 774.17-775.1 (CG 106-107); trans. Cooper 106: "As for the sixth day, some patients may suffer a crisis in it, but this is accompanied by severe symptoms, and with very serious danger. The crisis that occurs in it is not trustworthy, nor does it finish." Cf. sections 11 and 14 below.

6 Added according to the correct reading in MS Tehran. Cf. following note.

7 Cf. Galen, K 774.13-17 (CG 104-107); trans. Cooper 104, 106: "The species of the critical days derive from the fact that I have never seen anyone who suffered a crisis in the twelfth and the sixteenth day of the illness…"). MS Tehran lists the thirteenth day instead of the sixteenth. See as well section 12 below.

8 The text is cumbersome but clear, i.e., the body is strong enough to overcome the disease, but not on the first try. This section, next to 5-7, does not seem to be a summary, but an expansion of the first paragraph of *Critical Days* (K 769.1-770.6; CG 96-97), with additions from other works, such as *Aphorisms* and *Prognosis*. We thank Vivian Nutton for this comment.

that he maintained when he was healthy, little by little. [It consists in] riding horses, sitting on a litter that moves on the camel carrying it,[9] going to the bathhouse, drinking appropriate beverages and eating fitting food, such as the meat of pullets and fish that frequent rocks.

[7] However, with regard to diseases that have set in in such a way that the patient is not confident [of full recovery], then the regimen must be similar to the regimen of the ill. This regimen will then prevent a relapse if the disease that has abated is mild. For mild diseases that are not accompanied by any malicious, bad symptoms can be prevented from relapsing. If the disease is severe and malicious, and then the patient is given a regimen like that he maintained while ill, the relapse of the disease is such that there is no near and present danger. But if he is given a regimen by which he is not fortified against it, its relapse is dangerous.

[8] Some of the signs of the crisis are due to the organ that is expelling the residue, for example, the[10] attraction upwards of the abdominal wall; others are due to the organ that is conveying and moving forth the residue, for example, difficulty in breathing (shortness of breath); yet others are due to the organ that receives the residue, for example, lachrymation, headache, delirium, lethargy, heaviness in the temples, neck pain, palpitation, and shivers; still others are due to the residue itself, for example the flash that a person may see, and the darkness of vision.[11]

[9] Finding the true nature of the critical days is difficult and burdensome, because it is difficult to perceive the expiry of the disease and to grasp it. For the crisis sometimes extends for many days. For this reason,[12] some people say that the first day is the crisis day, I mean, the day on which the crisis began to develop. Others say that the second day is the crisis day; it is the day on which the greatest span of time of the crisis is discerned.[13] Still

---

9 The first set of instructions in MS Tehran is quite different: "[It consists in] riding stallions and sitting on stallions and seats that are in motion…". The reading of MS Princeton, *bakr*, "young camel", is possibly an error (in dictation) and should be corrected to *baqar*, "cow" or "ox".

10 K 775.10-12: "attraction upwards of the abdominal wall" (انجذاب مراق البطن إلى فوق); cf. CG101, l.4: انجذاب مراق الشراسيف إلى فوق (what is under the hypochondrium contracts; trans. Cooper, CG 100).

11 Similar and other symptoms are noted by Galen (K 771.10-772.3; CG 98-101); however the link between specific symptoms and organs is missing in Galen.

12 Following MS Tehran; MS Princeton probably intends the same, but the copyist has probably skipped a word. The text should read وإن كان ذلك كذلك.

13 Cf. Galen (K 779.5): εἰς ἣν ὁ πλεῖστος χρόνος τῆς κρίσεως ἀφίκετο; ed. and trans. Cooper (CG 112-115;): وهو الذي يكون فيه أكثر زمان البحران (that in which the time of the crisis is of

others say that the third day is the crisis day; it is the day on which the disease terminates. The true crisis day is the day on which all of the signs of the crisis come together; less[14] than that [for the purposes of] counting the critical days is the one on which the signs of the crisis diminish by one or two signs (i.e., four or five signs are present).[15] The day on which the disease turns (i.e. changes direction), for example, on [that day] the crisis will not be complete. It is the day on which three signs of the crisis are present, and three are absent.

[10] The crisis occurs more often on some of the critical days; these are the good (auspicious) days, like the seventh day. The crisis comes on this day for most patients. It is a good crisis, complete, sure of outcome, safe from danger. Warning of its [approach] has been given already, for the fourth day warns by means of a change that takes place on it in the concoction of the urine, or in the spittle, or in the excrement, or in activity with regard to appetite, sensation, intellect and sleep.[16]

[11] The crisis occurs less often on others, and these are the bad days, for example the sixth day. The crisis occurs then for only a few patients. It is a bad crisis, not complete, not clear, unsure of outcome, and not safe from danger.[17]

[12] On the other [days] there will not be a crisis, i.e, the twelfth day or sixteenth.[18]

[13] Some people call any sudden change that occurs in the patient a crisis.[19] Others call a crisis only the change in the direction of recovery. Still others call a crisis the agitation that precedes the disengagement,[20] especially the doctors,[21] since it is their task to investigate the things themselves, and especially of the dialecticians [whose task is] to investigate the

---

the greatest extent). Note that the term زمان is found in the Tehran MS, contrary to the Princeton MS which has وقت.

14 "less" (أقلّ); i.e. in the sense of less certain or decisive for beginning the count of days.

15 Cf. Galen, K 780.2-11 (CG 116-117); see as well K 782.16-783.10 (CG 120-123).

16 Cf. Galen, K 784.5-16 (CG 124-125). Instead of "sleep", Galen refers to "any other change of that sort" (ἤ τινος ἄλλου τοιούτου σαφὴς ἐγένετο μεταβολὴ which is rendered by Ḥunayn as: أو في غير ذلك ممّا أشبهه (trans. Cooper 124: "or in anything else of that sort").

17 Cf. Galen, K 791.16 (CG 136-137); see as well section 3 above and 14 below.

18 Cf. Galen (K 788.1; CG 130-131); see as well section 3 above.

19 MS Tehran reads here: "People disagree about the change that comes about in the disease. Some of them call..."

20 Literally, "what precedes the disengagement in terms of agitation". MS Tehran reads: "Still others call a crisis the preceding agitation". Cf. Galen, K 788.12-16 (CG 132-133).

21 "the doctors" is missing in MS Tehran.

correctness of the terms, and their normal usage.[22] So also is it especially [the task of] those charged with upholding[23] the Greek language and the rhetoricians[24]—that is the art that seeks to convince[25]—they are charged with investigating the terms that have come to be used habitually and the foreign terms.[26]

[14] When the crisis that occurs on the sixth day tends towards a more ruinous condition, then, beforehand, on the fourth day,[27] shortness of breath, chills, shivers, dwindling of strength, uneven sweating in the body, and the elimination of unripe materials will be present.[28]

[15] On some of the crisis days, the crisis comes constantly,[29] but on others it will come only rarely. For others, the situation is in between. As for the days on which the crisis comes constantly, some belong to the first class of critical days, that is (*bi-manzila*) the seventh day and the fourteenth; some belong to the second class, that is the ninth day, the nineteenth, and the twentieth; others belong to the third class, that is, the seventeenth day, and the fifth; yet others belong to the fourth class, that is, the fourth day, the third, and the eighteenth.

---

22 "and especially of the dialecticians [whose task is] to investigate the correctness of the terms, and their normal usage" (وإجرائها مجاريها): cf. Galen (K 789.5-6): διαλεκτικοῦ μὲν γὰρ ὑπὲρ ὀνομάτων ὀρθότητος σκοπεῖσθαι (for it is the task of the dialectician to investigate the matter of the correctness of the names); trans. Ḥunayn (CG 133): وذلك أنّ من شأن صاحب المنطق أن يبحث عن استقامة وضع الأسماء; trans. Cooper 132: "This is because it is appropriate for the logician to investigate whether names have been assigned properly".

23 *Iqāma*, omitted in MS Tehran, which later supplies *taqwīm* in its place. Clearly the grammarians are intended here.

24 MS Princeton transcribes the Greek term: *aṣḥāb al-rūṭūrīqā*, while MS Tehran employs the Arabic equivalent, *al-khuṭabāʾ*.

25 This parenthetical remark is omitted in MS Tehran.

26 Cf. Galen (K 789.5-6): ῥητόρων δὲ καὶ γραμματικῶν, εἰ σύνειθες τοῖς Ἕλλησι τοὔνομα (and [it is appropriate] for rhetoriticians and grammarians [to investigate] whether the word is customary with the Greeks; cf. trans. Ḥunayn (CG 133): ومن شأن النحوي والبليغ أن يبحث هل جرت العادة باستعمال الاسم أم لا; trans. Cooper 132: "and it is appropriate for the grammarian and the rhetorician to investigate whether the word conforms to proper usage".

27 MS Tehran begins this passage: "It is characteristic of a change towards a worse condition that it come about on the sixth day, and that it be preceded by..." (see the previous discussion).

28 Cf. Galen, K 785.18-786.4 (CG 126-127).

29 "constantly" (دائما); i.e. frequently.

[16] As for the days on which the crisis comes only rarely,[30] some belong to the first class, i.e., the fifth day and the sixth; others belong to the second class, i.e., the eighth day and the fifteenth day; still others belong to the third class, i.e., the twelfth day. As for the days whose status is midway between these, they are the thirteenth day and the sixteenth day.[31]

[M1] Marginal note: Chief among them with regard to rarity is that which he put in the third class, exemplified by the twelfth [day]. This is an incongruity in the nature of the days on which the crisis will always be. He made the first class of them chief in this regard [frequency]. You may find an indication of what I have said in that Galen stated, "As far as I have seen, the crisis never comes on the twelfth [day]". As for the sixth, it belongs to what he placed in the first class, since the crisis rarely falls on it. He mentioned that the bad crisis frequently falls on it. They were ordered in this way only because he made that belonging to the first class on which the crisis rarely falls adjacent to the extremity of the class in which the crisis always falls; so it is most [frequently] found of the rare [cases]. He made the end of the class of the rare [sort] those that are only infrequently found. Thus the critical days, those that are frequently found and those that are rarely found, are arranged in this way according to their frequency of occurrence. The most frequent is first in the group [and] the rarest is at the end of the group.

[17] For some people, the onset of illness is the moment when discomfort is sensed. For others, it is when the person takes to bed. People differ with regard to being bedridden. Some lie down before the illness sets in because of their feebleness, and the weakness of their soul. Others do this after the illness has come to be, on account of a strong soul and good forbearance and ability to cope. Yet others are prevented from taking to bed because they are busy with worldly affairs; they lie down only at the end of the illness. For some people the onset of the disease is the moment in which they sense the distress of the disease.[32]

[18] For some patients, the disease sets in all at once. It is not preceded by any signs that indicate it. For others, the disease does not set in all at once, but [only] after[33] they are discomforted and the symptoms of the disease

---

30 Here MS Princeton inserts a long marginalium, printed below as [M1]. The beginning of this sentence in MS Tehran is slightly different: "As for the days on which the crisis hardly comes at all, but only rarely, that [group] falls into three grades..."

31 Galen, K 792 -793.9 (CG 138-141) discusses the crisis and non-crisis days up to the twentieth day, but does not classify them as precisely as here.

32 Cf. Galen, K 795.18-796.8 (CG 144-145).

33 "after they are discomforted" (بعد ما ينالهم الأذى); Galen, K 796.19-797.1 states that many diseases begin accompanied by shivering fits and pains (ἅμα ῥίγεσιν, ἢ σὺν ἀλγήμασιν);

are brought forth. Once they are discomforted, then fever will begin in them afterwards.[34]

[19] The onset of the disease is of two sorts: either in view of nature, and that is the onset that is said to be discerned by reason; or else it is in view of sensation, which is the one recognized and according to which one must act.[35]

[20] When the crisis falls on two days without being preceded by a warning day, one must solve for the critical day by reasoning on the basis of cycles, the nature of the day, the number of critical days, and the moment of crisis.[36]

[21]There are three moments in which the crisis takes place. One of these is the moment of the fever's paroxysm, the second the moment of evacuation, and the third, the moment of relief.[37] If these moments are present on the same day, we say that that is the critical day. If they take place on two days, then only the day about which the warning day gave warning ought to be called the critical day. If the crisis takes place on two days, then, should most of the critical symptoms be found on the first of them, but only some of them on the second day, then some of the crisis should be given to the second day. But if these symptoms are found altogether on the two days, then the crisis applies to both of them.[38]

[22] The critical days after the twentieth day are, according to the adherents of Hippocrates and Galen,[39] the twenty-fourth, the twenty-seventh,

---

cf. Ḥunayn (CG 147): إما بنافض وإما بوجع قويّ; trans. Cooper 146: either accompanied by a tremor or a strong pain.

34 Cf. Galen, K 796.18-797.1 (CG 144-147).

35 The author means to say that the onset of the disease can be viewed in two ways: 'by nature' or theoretically, whereby we conclude that the disease began at a certain moment, even though no symptoms are yet present; and empirically. Note, however, that Galen, K 797.10-801.4 (CG 146-153), polemicises with the Sophists for whom the time of the illness is known through thought and reason alone. MS Tehran adds here: "The indications, by way of example. Some indicate the crisis, and the preceding day warns by means of an auspicious indication. Some indicate its appearance, and [they are] the critical symptoms, tremors and sweat. Some do not indicate any danger; they are the unusual (*gharība*) symptoms. As for its completion, it is the relief from the fever (?). As for that which [occurs?] at its onset (i.e. of the completion), it [indicates] its heading towards relief. As for that which indicates confidence [in full recovery?], it is all of them together".

36 Cf. Galen, K 810.3-8 (CG 168-169).

37 "relief" (التخلّص من المرض); i.e. that one is relieved from the illness; i.e. that the illness is over; cf. Galen, K 810.18: τὸ τέλος αὐτὸ τῆς κρίσεως (the end (cessation) of the crisis); cf. trans. Ḥunayn (CG 171): انقضاء البحران; trans. Cooper 170: "the resolution of the crisis".

38 Cf. Galen, K 810.16-811.9 (CG 170-171).

39 MS Princeton adds: "the twentieth day".

the thirty-first, the thirty-fourth, the thirty-seventh, and the fortieth. But according to the adherents of Archigenes, they are the twenty-first day, the twenty-eighth, the forty-second, the forty-fifth, and the forty-eighth.[40]

[23] From among the cycles of the stars, three cycles are correlates [of the cycles of critical days],[41] I mean, the cycle of the moon, the cycle of the sun, and the cycle of Saturn.[42] Hippocrates recorded the fortieth day, the sixtieth day, the eightieth day, and the hundred and twentieth day among the critical days.[43]

[M2][44] Regarding the text, in this [i.e. first?] book, but not where he mentioned the stars in the third (book??) did he mention Saturn and ...among the [zodiacal] signs which the author of the Summaries mentioned here in book two. The author of the Summaries said afterwards, in book three, as in the case of (*manzila*) the fourteen, which is taken in analogy to the moon when it is on its diameter [diametrically opposed to the sun, full moon, half cycle], that is, six months when taken in analogy to the sun (14 days of lunar cycle analogous to 6 months in solar cycle), and fourteen [years] when taken in analogy to the cycle of Saturn.

[24] Exiting the disease may [continue from the crisis] up to the fourteenth day, with great effort,[45] but with a moderate effort it aims for the fortieth day. But only rarely will it be with an effort and [yet] after the fortieth [day], and only in the diseases whose termination exceeds [the usual period]; and it is those in which the crisis lasts for three days.

[25] Galen said that the one who wishes to know beforehand about the crisis should be cognizant of Hippocrates' *Prognosis*.[46] He should also be experienced and skilled in the actual practice on patients. He may know it [also] from the pulse of the arteries and its rules.[47]

[26] Some signs indicate rescue and safety, others perdition and demise, yet others danger, and still others the ripening of the disease.[48]

[27] The signs that indicate safety are that the strength [of the body] is strong, the breathing easy, the illness is light upon the body, and the pulse

40 Cf. Galen, K 815.17-816.11 (CG 170-171).

41 MS Tehran reads here: "The correlated cycles are three..."

42 Text missing in Galen.

43 Cf. Galen, K 817.9 (CG 170-171).

44 This marginalium, found like the others in MS Princeton, is cut off in left margin.

45 The "effort" (*jihād*) spoken of here is the exertion of "nature" (the bodily faculties) to rid itself of the illness.

46 Cf. Galen, K 818.9-17 (CG 184-185).

47 Cf. Galen, K 818.1-7 and 818.16 (CG 182-185).

48 Cf. Galen, K 819.8-9 (CG 184-185).

nice and good.

[28] The signs that indicate perdition are poor breathing, a heaviness of the body, and a bad pulse. The signs of danger are cold sweat; and the signs of ripening are ripe urine.

[29] If the error that befalls in the matter of patients is of a small magnitude, an incomplete crisis is brought about thereby on the seventh day. But if it is of a great magnitude, it is brought about thereby on the ninth day or on the eleventh day.[49] The error may be due to the physician, it may be due to the patient, and it may be due to his family[50] and servants; and it may be due to exterior events, that is, noise, a quarrel with neighbors,[51] and bad news, for example, news of a disturbance or of a fire; or the bringing of sad news concerning family, property, or friend.[52] A crisis that leads back to safety comes late, but in the case of fatal diseases it comes early.[53] It will be on the fifth day, if the illness is acute, its paroxysms fall on odd days, and the error in connection to the patient was great;[54] or on the sixth day, if the situation is the opposite.

[30] For some diseases it is possible to know from the very outset the type of each one, and what will be the outcome at the end; for example, tertian fever in which the signs of ripening are clear.[55] It will come to an end on the fourth day. For others it is not possible to get knowledge about anything concerning these two things [type, outcome], such as tertian fever, when there are two fevers, and on the first days symptoms are discerned which indicate

---

49 MS Tehran adds here: "If the error is on the part of the patient, then, with regard to illnesses that are not dangerous, they will be long-term and their dissipation will take a long time. But diseases that are dangerous lead to perdition. That which terminates in relief is [not!] dangerous."

50 Om. MS Tehran.

51 MS Tehran adds: "and the sound of war". MS Tehran omits "concerning family, property, or friend".

52 Cf. Galen, K 822.8-17, 824.1-12; CG 190-197.

53 Galen, K 828.13 merely states that safe illnesses usually last longer because of errors (ἐπὶ τοῖς ἁμαρτήμασι); cf trans. Ḥunayn (CG 203): إذا عرض فيها عارض; trans. Cooper 202: "if an accident occurs in them"; see as well CG 190, n.397. MS Tehran's formulation is as follows: "Its occurrence will come early. But with regard to illnesses that are not dangerous, their crises come late."

54 In place of the last phrase MS Tehran reads, "and the danger is great".

55 This passage is very different in MS Tehran: "For some diseases it is possible to know from the very outset the type of each one, and what will be the outcome at the end; for example, tertian fever, when there is a fever that is manifest (*tabīnu*), but in the first days the signs of ripening were not manifest. For others, its species is known, but it is not known how it will end up, such as prolonged phlegmatic fever. "

that the disease has not ripened. For yet others, neither its type nor the outcome at which it will end can be known, for example, phlegmatic fever.

[31] Some diseases are safe, they come to an end on the fourth day, and the symptoms of ripening are clear from the first day. Whoever has a disease that is like this should be given a very fine and light regimen. Others are fatal, and they will come to an end on the fourth day. Still others are safe, but they are accompanied by symptoms that indicate that the illness has not ripened; sometimes it is accompanied by symptoms that indicate that it will be prolonged. If the two characteristics are found together, it is a disease that will last a long time, and the person who suffers from it should be given a thick regimen. But if one of them is found, I mean only a symptom that indicates that the disease has not ripened, then it is a disease that will not last for long. The person who suffers from it should be given a regimen that is less thick.[56]

[32] If the signs of ripening are clear on the fourth day, then the crisis will be in the seventh day; if they are clear on the seventh day, then the crisis will come on the fourteenth day; if they are clear on the fourteenth day, then the crisis will come either on the seventeenth day, the eighteenth day, the twentieth day, or on the twenty-first day. The seventeenth day will give warning about one of these three [other] days.[57]

[33] If the disease is prolonged, and signs are discerned that it has not ripened, or that it will be [even more] prolonged; then, if those signs are discerned on the seventh day, the indication is that it will terminate on the fourteenth day. But if they are discerned on the eleventh day, then the disease will terminate after the twentieth day; and if they are discerned on the seventeenth day, then the disease will terminate on the fortieth day.[58]

[34] The summaries[59] of the first book of Galen's tract *On Critical Days* are finished. Praise to God, and His prayers on his prophet Muhammad and his pure family.[60]

---

56 This statement is missing in Galen. Cf., however, the more general statement in Galen, bk. 2, K 885.16-886.9 (CG 296-299), where he remarks that if one anticipates the crisis on the third or fourth day and the patient is a strong young man, one may withhold food until the fourth day, or even the seventh day. However, if the crisis occurs between the seventh day and the eleventh or fourteenth, one may not withhold food from him.

57 Cf. K 836.3-837.14 (CG 218-221). MS Tehran reads for the last sentence, "will give warning about one of these two days".

58 Cf. K 838.7-839.9 (CG 222-225).

59 MS Tehran adds: "of the Alexandrians".

60 For the final sentence MS Tehran displays: "Much Praise to God alone."

[35] In the name of God, the Compassionate, the Merciful. The summaries of the second book of Galen's book *On Critical Days*.

Three things cause people to differ with regard to the issue of crisis.[61] The first is that it is difficult and toilsome to establish the beginning of the disease.[62] The second is that error may occur either on the part of the physician or on the part of the patient.[63] The third is that the crisis may last for many days.[64]

[36] Some days are critical days, some days are warning days, and some days lie in between. The true[65] critical days are the fourth, the seventh, the eleventh, the fourteenth, the seventeenth, and the twentieth. The days that give warning of the crisis are the fourth, the eleventh, and the fourteenth.[66] The days that lie in between are the third, the fifth, the sixth, the thirteenth, and the fifteenth.[67].

[37] The tetrads of the critical days differ with regard to their number.[68] The first tetrad and the second tetrad overlap (*mawṣūlayn*); the second tetrad and the third tetrad are counted separately; the third and fourth are consecutive, and the fourth and the fifth also overlap, since the fifth terminates on the seventeenth day. So also do the fifth and sixth overlap.[69]

[38] The ancients were all in agreement about the critical days up to the fourteenth day. However, they disagreed about the days after it. That is to say, one group of them claimed that the critical days after the fourteenth day are the seventeenth day, the twentieth day, the twenty-fourth day,[70] the

61 MS Tehran displays: "The causes for disagreement in the views of people concerning the issue of the crisis are three." A marginal note in MS Princeton reads: "Three things that are difficult to establish: The beginning of the disease, the occurrence of an error, and the length of the crisis."

62 The problem of establishing the beginning of a disease has been discussed into detail in bk. 1; K 795.9-797.16 (CG 142-149).

63 Cf. Bk. 1, section 29. MS Tehran adds "or on the part of the servants or on account of external events".

64 Cf. Bk. 1, section 9.

65 Om. T.

66 Cf. Galen, K 845.10-16 (CG 234-235); see as well K 875.15-876.5 (CG 282-283).

67 Galen, K 847.9-11 (CG 238-239), mentions the third, the fifth, the sixth, and the ninth as falling between the critical days.

68 "with regard to their number" means here, "the way they are counted". When tetrads overlap, the second begins on the last day of the first, so that the sum total of the two tetrads is seven, not eight; here we have 4 + 2nd=7, 7+ 3rd=**11**; 11 + 4th=**14**; 14 +5th =**17**; 17 + 6th =**20**. 7, 11, 14, 17, and 20 are all critical days.

69 This section is not found in Galen.

70 MS T has here instead the twenty-first day.

twenty-seventh day, the thirty-first day, the thirty-fourth day, the fortieth day, the sixtieth day,[71] the eightieth day, and the hundred-and-twentieth day. Another group claims that[72] they are the eighteenth day, the twenty-first day, the twenty-fifth day, the twenty-eighth, the thirty-second day, the thirty-fifth day, the forty-second day, and the forty-eighth.[73]

[39] The writings [composed by] Hippocrates called "Epidemics" consist of seven books.[74] Two of these books are authentic [*ṣāḥīḥān*], there is no doubt about them; they are the first and the third. There is doubt concerning three of them; they are the second, the fourth, and the sixth.[75] Two are fabrications and forgeries;[76] they are the fifth and the seventh.[77]

[40] If the illnesses are such that the crisis continues for many days, we must learn about the affair of the crisis from the beginning of the illness, from the day that warns of the crisis, and from the movements of the illness's paroxysms.

[41] Some crises are well-defined; they are the ones which come about and terminate in one day. Others are not well-defined; they are the ones that last for many days.

[42] The exit from the disease is of three sorts: by ripening and dissolution,[78] if the thing that activates the disease[79] is worn out over time; by evacuation, if all of the matter that activates the disease is expelled outwards in its entirety; by an abscess or an ulcer, if the thing is pushed to a non-noble organ.

[43] Some chronic illnesses terminate by ripening and dissolution; for others, the termination is all at once, and that is when the illness moves at the end of the affair with an acute motion.[80] Also, for some chronic diseases, the crisis lasts for many days. For others, the crisis begins and ends on one day.

---

71 Om. T.

72 T adds here "the critical days that come after the fourteenth day".

73 T has here instead the forty-fourth day. Cf. Galen, K 853.7-854.5 (CG 246-247). Referring to Hippocrates, Galen distinguishes between two classes of critical days; the last days mentioned representing these two classes are the fortieth and forty-second.

74 T calls *On Epidemics* "a book" (in the singular, *kitāb*), and its seven sections, *maqālāt*.

75 Our translation is according to the supralinear note in the Princeton MS which reads والسادس instead of: والسابع. T agrees with the corrected reading of P, i.e., books 2, 4, and 6.

76 T uses one word only, which does not appear in P: *manḥūla*, "spurious".

77 Cf. Galen, K 859.15-18 (CG 258-259).

78 Om T.

79 T has "the humour which is the cause".

80 T expresses the same idea but formulates it more concisely. Instead of "the termination is all at once, and that is when the illness moves at the end of the affair with an acute motion", T has: "the termination is all at once, at the end, with a fast motion".

[44] The natures of critical days are of two natures. Some are true criticals, others are false criticals. The true criticals are called critical by nature; they are the fourth day, and the seventh, fourteenth, and twentieth. The false criticals are the third, fifth, ninth and thirteenth.[81]

[45] Knowledge of the critical days is useful in two ways. It is useful for foreknowledge[82] of the crisis. For we know crises only from the signs and indications that warn about them. It is useful [also] for calculating nourishment.[83] For if we know the day on which the illness terminates, we may calculate the nourishment accordingly.[84]

[46] Hippocrates took note of the days critical by nature—and they are the true critical days—and the days that fall between the true critical days.[85] That is, he mentioned them in the *Aphorisms* and in the *Prognosis*; and he mentioned in the first book of *Epidemics* those that are critical days by nature, and the days that fall between them.[86]

[47] Some of those days that fall between them[87] fall on even [numbered days], and some fall on odd ones. Those that fall on even ones are the sixth, the eighth, the tenth, the twentieth, and the twenty-eighth;[88] those that fall on odd ones are the third, the fifth, and the ninth.[89]

[48] Some of the cycles of critical days are tetrads [literally: in four four],

---

81 Again, T has the same idea expressed more succinctly: "The nature of critical days is two-fold. That is, some of them are critical by nature, like the fourth, seventh, fourteenth, and twentieth. Others are only thought to be critical, such as the third, the fifth, the seventh, and the thirteenth."

82 Accepting the marginalium in P, which corrects *sāʾir* to *sābiq*. For T's term *taqdima maʿrifa*, see table on p. 30.

83 T reads here: "to be informed about the determination of the plan of the regimen".

84 Cf. Galen, K 869.10-13 (CG 272-273).

85 "and they are the true critical days—and the days that fall between the true critical days" is omitted in T.

86 Cf. Galen, K 868.11-17 (CG 270-271). Note that referrring to Hippocrates, Galen speaks about (true) critical days as being twofold: some increase by series of four and some by sevens (here referring to Hippocrates' *Aphorisms*). Additionally he mentions (referring to Hippocrates' *Epidemics*) the days occurring between them. T has here instead, "But as for the first book of the *Aphorisms*, he spoke there not only about the critical days, but also about the days that lie between them."

87 "that fall between them" om. T.

88 "and the twenty-eighth" om. T.

89 Cf. Galen, K 871.10-13 (CG 276-277). Quoting from Hippocrates' *Epidemics*, Galen also mentions the thirty-fourth, fortieth, sixtieth, eightieth, and hundred-twentieth day amongst the even days, while amongst the odd days he also mentions the seventh, eleventh, seventeenth, twenty-first, twenty-seventh, and thirty-first day.

others are heptads, others are twenty [icosads]. Those that are in fours are the days that end in the twentieth; those that are in sevens are from the twentieth [with the days overlapping as explained above] to the thirty-fourth; and those that are in twenties are the days from the fortieth to the sixtieth.[90]

[49] The causes of discrepancy in the matter of critical days are many. One of them is ignorance with regard to the two natures of critical days, I mean, those that are critical days by nature and those that are false.[91] The second is that their investigator restricts himself to theoretical reasoning, without [taking into account] experience.[92] The third is that when a person sees that a crisis falls once upon one of the days, he judges that it is one of the critical days; he does not anticipate [any more], in order to see whether there will be a crisis on it [i.e., that particular day] at other times or not. The fourth is that the person does not know that the critical days and the types of crises may be concurrent, like epidemic diseases.[93] The concurrence[94] may be with regard to the diseases, with regard to the types of crises, or with regard to the critical days.

[50] As for the diseases,[95] at some times they are burning fevers, at others tertian fevers, and at yet others quartan fevers.[96] As for the types of crisis,[97] the crises will at times be [in the form of] nosebleeds, at others sweating, at

90 Carrying on with the explanation given above, 7+7+6=20, 20+7=27, 27+7=34.

91 T is more concise: "those that are thus by nature and so those that are [mistakenly] thought to be [so]."

92 Cf. Galen, K 872.11-14 (CG 278-279). Galen merely mentions two kinds of critical days, without any qualification; according to Cooper, CG 270, n. 822, these are days by series of four and by seven. However, following Galen, K 868.11-17 (cf. section 46), it seems clear to us that these two kinds are the days that are critical by nature (i.e. by series of four and by seven) and those that are false, i.e. the intermediate days.

93 *wāfid*, "epidemic", or perhaps "syndemic". T speaks about the fact that he does not know the *fuṣūl* (periods) of the critical days and the *jihāt* (directions) of the crises.

94 "concurrence" (*wufūd*): T speaks, once again, about *fuṣūl*.

95 Cf. T: "As for those (i..e *fuṣūl* (periods) of the diseases."

96 From the "The fourth" in [49] to here, T has something completely different: "The fourth is that the person does not know about the periods (*fuṣūl*) of the crisis and the directions (*jihāt*) of the crises. With regard to illnesses, the periods may be on the part of the crises and on the critical days. But as for that which is in the disease [periods that have to do with the course of the illness and not with crises], they may produce in this [lapse of] time burning fevers, and in another time, tertian fever, and in yet another [time], quartan fever."

97 T speaks about the *fuṣūl* (periods) of the *anḥā* (directions) of the crises.

yet others vomiting. As for the critical days,[98] some will be at this time on the seventh day, others will be at another time, on the tenth day, yet others at a different time, on the eleventh day.

[51] Some days are critical only, and they are the seventh day, the fourteenth, and the twentieth. Others are jointly critical and warning, and they are the fourth day, the eleventh, and the seventeenth. Yet others fall in the middle, and they are the third, the fifth,[99] and the thirteenth.

[52] The way of reasoning with regard to the days is in this way: for the days before day twenty, the first two weeks are computed in a way that distinguishes among them between the first and second week[s]; but the third week is computed along with the second week in a way that it overlaps with it.[100] But as for the days that are after twenty, the first two weeks are again computed in such a way that distinguishes between them, so that the two of them end on day thirty-four [20 + 14]. The third week overlaps with the second week, ending on day forty.

[53] There are three cycles. One of them is a half-cycle ["cycle of a half"];[101] it is the cycle of tetrads, because when four is multiplied, there results eight, twelve, and sixteen. The other is the full cycle, and it is the cycle of heptads, because when seven is multiplied, the results are fourteen, twenty-one, twenty-eight, thirty-five, and forty-two. The third cycle is a fuller[102] cycle than that, and it is the cycle of twenties, because when twenty is multiplied the results are forty, sixty, eighty, and one hundred and twenty.[103]

[M3] Regarding this text: We must therefore make a division that was not required of us beforehand. We must add the distinct parts one to the other. That will be when we have divided that thing that is categorized as quantity into large parts. The division should not exceed the limit, to the point where there are very many parts, and, therefore, the quantity that is suited for instruction is surpassed.[104]

[54] A division of the illnesses must be made that is not in accordance with the critical days, otherwise it will be without limit; nor [should it be]

---

98 T speaks about the *fuṣūl* (periods) of the critical days

99 T adds "and the ninth".

100 I.e., one day on (in?) common, so that 20 days can form three heptads.

101 T adds: "(*al-jānib ʿan*) doubling" which could mean "half the quantity of double tetrads", and thus concord with Princeton, "One of them is a half-cycle ["cycle of a half"]; it is the cycle of tetrads".

102 T reads here "the fullest and most perfect".

103 K 879.3-879.7 (CG 286-287).

104 The marginal note refers to overdoing scholastic division into categories and subcategories, so that the whole thing becomes too cumbersome.

in accordance with their general classes, because that which is very distinct[105] does not relate one to the other. Rather, [it should be] commensurate with their movements [rate of progress of the disease].[106]

[55] So we say that some illnesses are of the utmost acuity and swiftness; others are [merely] acute; yet others fall short of acute diseases, falling within the chronic; still others are chronic, of long duration. Among the illnesses that are of the utmost acuity, some are at the ultimate extreme of acuity, i.e., continuous fevers that terminate after four days, while some are extreme,[107] i.e., burning fevers that abate in seven days. Among acute illnesses, some[108] are of extreme acuity, and they are those that terminate within fourteen days, while others are of a general acuity, and they are those that terminate within twenty days.[109] Among the illnesses that fall within [the range of] acute to chronic, some are ongoing, while others have paroxysms. Among chronic illnesses, some terminate within two months, others within seven months, still others within seven years, yet others within fourteen years.[110]

---

105 "is very distinct"; lit. made distinct by many distinctions.

106 Cf. K 881.15-883.1 (CG 290-295). The meaning seems to be this: theory has determined sets of critical days, and it has also classified fevers as hectic, tertian, etc. However, when it comes to practice, one should not rely upon these theoretical divisions, but rather pay attention to the course of each illness. T has here instead, "A division of the illnesses must be made that is not commensurate with the critical days, because they are not [precisely?] defined, nor also [commensurate] with their generic periods, because some of them do not bear a relation to the others [or: do not connect to the others], as the distinction between them is powerful. Instead, their division must be in accord with their movements."

107 The MS has the following marginal note: " that is, not the ultimate".

108 "of extreme acuity"; Galen does not speak of illnesses that are extremely acute but "acute in an exact way"; cf K 886.16: ἀκριβῶς μὲν ὀξὺ; Ḥunayn (CG 299) defines the Greek as فالذي يسمّى بهذا الاسم على الاستقصاء والحقيقة; trans. Cooper (CG 298): "that which is called by this name (i.e. "acute"), according to thorough investigation and in reality".

109 K 886.11-17; CG 298-299.

110 This passage is quite different in T: "Insofar [in T [55] continues the sentence begun in [54]] as we say that some diseases are very acute, they divide into two groups. One of them is at the utmost extremity of acuity, such as the continuous fever that is called 'synochous', which resolves [i.e. ends] on the fourth day. The other group is very acute, generally speaking [but not at the extreme], such as the burning fever that resolves on the seventh day. Others are acute, and they also divide into two groups. Some are acute at their end, and they are the illnesses whose resolution in general [takes place] up the fourteenth day, while others are acute, generally speaking, and they are those whose resolution will take place up to the twentieth day. Some illnesses are produced at the decline of acute illnesses, and they divide into two groups: some are permanent and some are recurrent (returning from time to time). Yet other illnesses are chronic, and

[56] Some illnesses are acute, namely those lasting for a short time; the person suffering from them is in danger[111] on their account, such as burning fever.[112] Others are of short duration, and they do not linger for long, but they are not accompanied by any danger, i.e., ephemeral fever. Still others fall out of [the category of] acute fevers into [that of] chronic ones; they are the ones whose movement from the beginning of the situation is slow, but then it becomes acute. Yet others are chronic; they are those whose movement from the beginning of the situation to the end is a mild movement.[113]

[57] Some illnesses are of the utmost extremity,[114] such that there is no extreme of acuity beyond them; they are those that terminate on the fourth day. The regimen of the patient in this case is that he should refrain from nourishment altogether. Others are very acute, but not of the ultimate acuity;[115] they are those that terminate on the seventh day. In that case, honey water alone should be employed. Others are of true [i.e., not extreme] acuity, and they are those that terminate within fourteen days. In their case, barley gruel, pure, just as it is,[116] should be employed.[117] Yet others occur from acuity to [the] chronic,[118] and others are long-lasting chronic [diseases]. Among these classes, some terminate within two months, oth-

---

their divisions are four. That is, for some the resolution (following our editorial emendation) is within two months, for others the resolution is within seven months, for others the resolution is within seven years, and for yet others the resolution is within fourteen years".

111 T adds "great danger".

112 T adds "that is called *qawsūs* (i.e. Greek καῦσος)".

113 K 887.5-10; CG 300-301. Galen does not define the type of fever accompanying these illnesses, but merely speaks of "fever". For this long, last sentence, beginning "Still others", T has: "Some are produced from the decline of acute illnesses. They are those whose movement at the beginning of the affair is slow, but then acute at the end. Others are acute. They are those whose movement from beginning to end is slow". Neither P nor T are very clear here, nor do either of them precisely convey Galen's remarks.

114 T adds, "of acuity", but then omits "such that there is no extreme of acuity beyond them".

115 Instead of "but not of the ultimate acuity" T exhibits "generally".

116 T makes the same statement, except that instead of "barley gruel, pure, just as it is", it has "pure barley water".

117 T has something quite different for "barley, pure, just as it is, should be employed" including accounts of categories not found in P, but unfortunately T itself is not transparent here.

118 This cumbersome formulation refers to a relapse; see [59] below and the note there referring to Galen. T, however, reads: "Yet others are acute, produced from the decline of the disease."

ers within seven months, yet others within seven years, still others within fourteen years. The regimen for these ought to be thick.[119]

[58] Among the illnesses that terminate on the fortieth day, some are those that terminate between the onset of the illness and the completion of fourteen days; others begin when it moves with acute movements during the critical days until after the twentieth [day]; yet others[120] take on this configuration afterwards. Their termination is either within seven months, or within seven years, or within fourteen years.

[59] Galen makes the limits of acute illnesses the fourteenth day and the fortieth day, and the limits of diseases that occur from acuity to [the] chronic the fortieth day and the sixtieth day.[121]

[60] Illnesses whose crisis comes on the twentieth day are either illnesses whose movements begin to move slowly, then, after the fourth or seventh day, move with acute movements; or illnesses for which the crisis comes on imperfectly.[122]

[61] The summaries of the second book of Galen's book *On Critical Days* are finished. Praise to God, Lord of the worlds, and His prayers for his prophet Muhammad and his pure family.

[62] In the name of God, the Compassionate, the Merciful.
God is responsible for (or: is the grantor of) success.
The summaries of the third book of Galen's book *On Critical Days*.[123]

The principles on the basis of which knowledge of the critical days is extracted are two: one is that which is true on the basis of that to which experience attests, and the other is that to which reason attests.[124]

[63] The moon has seven shapes; four are before fullness[125] and three

---

119 Cf. Galen, K 885.16-886.11 (CG 296-299). Note that the thick regimen for those that suffer from chronic illnesses is not mentioned by Galen.

120 The MS has the following marginal note: "that is, from among the illnesses that are chronic."

121 Cf. Galen, K 894.14-18 (CG 310-311), quoting Hippocrates. T has a somewhat clearer description of the relapse: "As for the illnesses that come about from the decline of other illnesses".

122 The text is possibly an elaboration on K 897.13-18 (CG 316-317).

123 "God is responsible...Critical Days" om. T.

124 Cf. CG 321: وهذه الأصول جنسان أحدهما يؤخذ من التجربة والآخر من القياس; trans. Cooper 320: "These principles are of two kinds: one is derived from experience, and the other from reason". Galen (K 900.5) merely states that these principles are of two kinds, without defining them.

125 The MS has the following marginal note: "before fullness and including it".

are after fullness. As for the four that are before the fullness, one is called in Greek *mēnoeidēs*, and it is the new moon and it is called sextile. The second is called in Greek *dikhotomos*, which means divided in half, and it is called quartile. The third is called in Greek *amphikurtos*, which means having two convexities [i.e., convex on each side], and it is called trine. The fourth is called in Greek *panselēnos*, and it is the fullness, the full moon, and it is called opposition. As for the three that are after fullness, they are the one possessing two[126] boundaries, the one divided in half, and the disappearance.[127]

[M4] I did not find the Greek names in the text.

[64] When the sun is overhead,[128] the season is summer. When it descends toward the direction of the south, it is the season of winter. When it is in Aries, the season is spring, and when it is in Libra, the season is autumn.[129]

[65] [Concerning] what occurs in the air from the visibility of the crescent to its disappearance: At the moment of conjunction very powerful and very long-lasting changes occur.[130] At fullness there are powerful changes but they are of short duration. At the halfway point there are great changes. When it takes on a convex shape there are weak changes, and at its disappearance the changes are negligible.[131]

[66] The visibility of the crescent may be swift or slow [i.e., of long or short duration after the last visibility of the waning moon], depending upon four causes; that is, at one time it will be seen on the second day [after last visibility], at another time it will be seen on the third day. The reason[s] for this may be its proper motion, or the difference in latitude, or on account of the moment of conjunction, or on account of the difference in latitude.[132]

---

126 Though it is correct that this shape has two boundaries, it is most likely a minor graphic error in the Arabic, and the intention is the one having two convexities mentioned earlier.

127 Cf. Galen, K 902.14-903.1 (CG 324-325). There are two Arabic terms for quarter moon, *dhū al-ḥaddatayn*, "possessing two boundaries", and *dhū al-ḥadabatayn*, "possessing two convexities [or: curvatures]". The second is more faithful to the Greek; but the two are orthographically similar in Arabic and easily confused.

128 Literally, "at the zenith", but this is not correct for Greece or Iraq.

129 Cf. Galen, K 903.13 (CG 326-327); no mention of the zodiac.

130 The beginning of this passage reads in T as follows: "That which we have learned from observation is that the change that comes about at the syzygies is very powerful and [very] slow."

131 Cf. Galen, K 904.9-16 (CG 328-329). Instead of "negligible," T has "weak".

132 A dittography in P; one of these should probably be *ikhtilāf al-manāẓir*, parallax. T has "on account of the anomalous motion of the zodiacal signs (*al-latī li-l-burūj*)", which makes no sense. If we correct *li-l-burūj* to *fī al-burūj* ("in the signs"), then we have another wording for the first cause, so T should also be emended so as to list the parallax,

[67] There are four heptads in the cycle of the moon. One is from the moment of its visibility until it is divided in half, and that is in Taurus and Leo at quadrature. The second [extends] until it becomes full moon, and that is in Scorpio and Aquarius at quadrature. The third [extends] until the moment that it is divided into two halves as it wanes, and it is in Aries and Cancer at quadrature. The fourth [extends] until its complete disappearance, and that is in Libra and Capricorn at quadrature.[133]

[68] The cycles of critical days: some critical cycles are daily, others monthly, others yearly. The daily ones are the fourth, the seventh, and the fourteenth. The monthly ones are the fortieth day and six months.[134] The yearly ones are seven years and fourteen years. The relation (*qiyās*) of the cycles to their analogues[135] follows in this way. Fourteen, when related to the cycle of the moon, is at its diameter (full moon), [and is] analogous to six months when related to the cycle of the sun and to the fourteen years when related to the cycle of Saturn (is one half of its orbit). Also, the seventh day in the lunar cycle is like a period of three months in the cycle of the sun and like seven years in the cycle of Saturn. According to this pattern also, the fourth day in the lunar cycle, when it is sextile, is the forty-fifth day of the cycle of the sun.

[69] The beginning of the diseases proceeds in two ways. One of them is the beginning that we see with our own eyes in the coming about of each one of them. The other is the beginning in which the air changes on account of the sun in each month, and on account of the moon[136] in each week.[137]

[70] That which compels the crisis in a disease to come earlier is precisely the great severity and difficulty of the disease.[138] The error that takes place is on the part of the physician, or on the part of the patient, on the part of

---

which is indeed a strong variable in this computation. Cf. Galen, K 906.7-907.5 (CG 320-323).

133 Cf. Galen, K 908.4-11 (CG 334-335), no mention of zodiac, but cf. K 910.16-911.8.

134 Cf. Galen, K 913.17-914.1 (CG 342-343). Galen only speaks of "periods of days, weeks, and of months".

135 Instead of analogues (*ashbāh*) T has "names".

136 T reads "on account of the weeks of the moon"; it is almost certainly a copyist's error, and we have deleted it from the edition.

137 Cf. Galen, K 915.11-16 (CG 344-347). Note that according to Galen (K 915.16), the sun causes the change in the air in the case of the whole year and the moon in the case of each month.

138 The beginning of the passage is somewhat unclear in T but it may be translated as follows: "It may be necessary (*qad yajibu ḍarūratan*, not very elegant) and it may be that the crises of the illnesses will come early, for two reasons; the first is the strength of the paroxysm, and the other…".

those attending him, family and especially servants, or on the part of external things that occur.[139] In the case of acute diseases, many critical days fall in the middle, I mean the third, the fifth, the sixth, and the ninth; but in the case of chronic diseases, they are few.[140]

[71] The expelling faculty in the body may sometimes move to expel the superfluity before [it is] fully ripened, on account of something that excites it, stimulating it to [do] this, either externally or internally. When externally, then it is on the part of the physician, the patient, his family and attendants, or the things that occur externally. When internally, it is [due to] the severity of the illness, the humour that is harmful, or a paroxysm of the fever.[141] All of these causes may move toward this with a slow motion after the ripening has intensified on account of its weakness.[142]

[72] The paroxysm of the fever moves every day in the case of phlegmatic fever; in the case of tertian fever, one day [yes], and one day not;[143] and in the case of quartan fever, one day [yes], two days not.[144]

[73] The adherents of Pythagoras claim that numbers are of two kinds. Some are odd, and they are masculine;[145] they are the third, the fifth, the seventh, and the ninth.[146] The crisis comes on the third [day] on account of the strength of the cycle and its compulsion; [on] the fifth, on account of the strength of nature;[147] [on] the seventh, on account of the moon; [on] the ninth, on account of the error that befalls, when it is great.[148] Others are even, and they are feminine;[149] they are the second, the fourth, the sixth, the eighth, and the tenth.

[74] The paroxysms of some diseases are continuous, as in the case of

---

139 Cf. Galen, K 916.4-11 (CG 346-347). Note that Galen does not specify those who attend the patient. See as well passage 71.

140 Cf. Galen, K 916.14 (CG 346-347). Note that Galen does not specify which days fall in the middle. T adds here, "The first cycle may be in the odd [days], and then it is the third, and it may be in the even [days], and then it is the fourth."

141 "of the fever" om. T.

142 Cf. Galen, K 918.8-13, 919.11-920.1 (CG 350-353).

143 For "one day [yes], and one day not" T has "every three days".

144 For "one day [yes], and two days not" T has "every four days". This is not in Galen as such but cf. K 921.4-9 (CG 354-355).]

145 Cf. Galen, K 922.18-923.1 (CG 356-357).

146 T adds "and the eleventh".

147 That is to say, the weakening of nature's strength, so that the crisis is delayed; T exhibits here, "the fatigue of nature".

148 T has instead,"[on] the ninth because of the sun and [on] the eleventh because of Saturn" . Cf. Galen, K 923.17-924.14 (CG 358-359).

149 Cf. Galen, K 923.1-2 (CG 356-357).Cf. Galen, K 922.18-923.1 (CG 356-357).

burning fever;[150] that is the one whose irruption and difficulty is day on, day off.[151] Others are of the genus of chronic illnesses, except that they move with acute movements, such as the fever compounded of phlegmatic fever and tertian fever. Yet others are lasting and continuous, such as blood fever; it is the one in which the fever follows a single pattern throughout all of its days.[152]

[75] The twentieth day belongs to the critical days for two reasons. One of them [and this is the first reason] is that diseases whose period is long and whose irruption and severity are on even days only terminate on one of the even days.[153] The second is that the weeks are not [composed of] seven full days, and that is because the year has three hundred and sixty-five and one-quarter days. The month has twenty-nine and one-sixth days. The week has six days, and one half and one-sixth.[154]

[76] Weeks have different ways of joining (literally: "relations") one to the other. The second week overlaps with the first week with a separate juncture, but the third enters the second with a continuous juncture.[155]

[77] The quarters also join to each other in different ways. The first quarter joins the second with a continuous juncture; the second joins the third with a separate juncture; the fourth joins the third with a continuous juncture; the fifth joins the fourth with a continuous juncture; the sixth joins the fifth with a continuous juncture.[156]

[78] Diseases belong to [different] classes. Some are acute, and their opposites are lingering[157] diseases that are slow of movement. Some are chronic, of long duration, and their opposites are diseases of short duration. Some linger for a long time and their opposite is ephemeral fever.[158]

[79] The summaries of the third book of Galen's book *On Critical Days* are complete, and the book is finished in its entirety. Praise to God, Lord of the worlds, and may He pray for his prophet Muhammad and his pure family.

---

150 T adds here as well "that is called *qawsūs*".

151 Here too T reads "every three days".

152 Cf. Galen, K 925.18-926.6 (CG 360-362).

153 Cf. Galen, K 928.11-12 (CG 364-365). Galen does not state that these diseases terminate on even days, but that their paroxysms occur on those days only: καὶ τοὺς παραξυσμοὺς αἱ ἀρτίαι λαμβάνουσιν; cf. trans. Ḥunayn (CG 365): ونوائب الحمّى فيه تكون في الأزواج.

154 Cf. Galen, K 929.3-12 (CG 366-367). T omits "one half".

155 Cf. Galen, K 937.13-938.1 (CG 380-383). The subject has been explained above, i.e. the famous "Galenic week".

156 Cf. Galen, K 938.1-12 (CG 380-383).

157 T has here "chronic".

158 This section does not appear in Galen as such, but cf. K 939.12-941.1 (CG 382-385).

CHAPTER 5

The Hebrew Version of Shimshon ben Shlomo

1 Manuscripts

The Hebrew translation by Shimshon ben Shlomo, about whom nothing at all is known except for the fact that he completed the translation of the Alexandrian Summaries on the eighth of August 1322,[1] is extant in the following MSS:[2]

1.1 MS Vienna Oesterreichische Nationalbibliothek Cod hebr. 29

(cat. Schwarz 174, 15)[3] (א); fols. 199b-204a; copied in 1452 in a Sephardic script. This manuscript is, except for some minor variations, identical with MS Parma, Biblioteca Palatina Cod. Parma 2919. [see page 94]

1.2 St. Petersburg RNL Heb. I 332 (ב)

Copied in a Sephardic script on 30 August 1322; no foliation. The MS has the following colophon on fol. 267b: "The translation of the Summaries of the Alexandrians of the books of Galen was completed on the eighth of Elul, 5082 (= 30 August 1322) by Shimshon ben Shlomo." [see page 95]

1.3 Paris Bibliothèque Nationale héb 1117 (ג)[4]

Fols. 256a-262a (Hebrew page numbers) or 249a-255a (Arabic numbers); copied in the 14th-15th centuries in a Sephardic script. The MS is incomplete and suffers from fading of the ink. From הנה יכלה ליום העשרים in section 23 the MS has been copied in a different script and becomes increasingly hard to read; the last words that could be read are יחסו העלות in section 24.

---

1 Cf. M. Steinschneider, *Die hebräischen Übersetzungen des Mittelalters und die Juden als Dolmetscher* (Berlin 1893, repr. Graz 1956), p. 654.

2 For the data of the following MSS we consulted the Online Catalog of Hebrew Manuscripts at The Institute of Microfilmed Hebrew Manuscripts in the National Library, Jerusalem, and the relevant printed catalogs. See as well Steinschneider, *Die hebräischen Übersetzungen des Mittelalters und die Juden als Dolmetscher*, pp. 654-655.

3 Cf. A.Z. Schwarz, *Die hebräischen Handschriften der Nationalbibliothek in Wien* (Leipzig 1925), p. 190.

4 Cf. H. Zotenberg (ed.), *Catalogues des Manuscrits hébreux et samaritains de la Bibliothèque Impériale* (Paris 1866), p. 205.

 | DOI 10.1163/9789004282223_006

1.4 *Paris, Bibliothèque Nationale héb 1118* (ד)[5]

Fols. 104a-108b; copied in a Sephardic script in the 15th century. An ever increasing section of the text on fol. 108a, חלושה (ch. 25) until fol. 108b: אמנם יהיו בשתי אלו התמונות (ch. 27) is missing. [see page 93]

1.5 *Parma, Biblioteca Palatina Cod. Parma 2919 (cat. Richler 1498)*[6] (ה)

No foliation; copied in the 15th century in a Byzantine script; illustration in the right and bottom margin of beginning of *ma'amar* two with Hebrew term: המבשרים.

1.6 *Paris, Bibliothèque Nationale héb. 884*[7]

Fols. 276a-279a; copied in the 15th century in a Byzantine script. The manuscript suffers from hiatuses (a large section from 14-18 is missing) and is riddled with errors, and its variants have as a rule not been incorporated in our edition. On the other hand, in one place at least (passage [26]) it displays the best reading.

The basic MS used for the edition is Paris BN 1117 until section 24, and from then on MS St. Petersburg. Variants of the other MSS mentioned above have been noted in the critical apparatus.

2 Sigla

א = MS Vienna Oesterreichische Nationalbibliothek Cod hebr. 29
א1 = Note in the margin(s) of MS Vienna Oesterreichische Nationalbibliothek Cod hebr. 29
ב = St. Petersburg RNL Heb. I 332
ב1 = Note in the margin(s) of St. Petersburg RNL Heb. I 332
ג = Paris Bibliothèque Nationale héb 1117
ד = Paris Bibliothèque Nationale héb 1118
ד1 Note in the margin(s) of MS Paris Bibliothèque Nationale héb 1118
ד2 Note above the line in MS Paris Bibliothèque Nationale héb 1118
ה = Parma, Biblioteca Palatina Cod. Parma 291
ה1 Note in the margin of MS Parma, Biblioteca Palatina Cod. Parma 291
ה2 = Note above the line in MS Parma, Biblioteca Palatina Cod. Parma 291

---

5 Cf. ibid., p. 206.

6 Cf. B. Richler, *Hebrew Manuscripts in the Biblioteca Palatina in Parma. Catalogue. Palaeographical and codicological descriptions: Malachi Beit-Arié* (Jerusalem 2001), p. 441.

7 Cf. Zotenberg, *Catalogues des Manuscrits hébreux et samaritains de la Bibliothèque Impériale*, p. 152.

3 Abbreviations

add = added by
ditt = dittography
inv = inverted by
om = omitted by

4 Vocabulary

Shimshon ben Shlomo was familiar with the Hebrew scientific idiom which was well-developed by the early fourteenth century. Nevertheless, some of his choices for medical terms are interesting and unique. Some of these will be noted presently. The philosophical terms used in Book Three are of special interest. The discussion of Pythagorean theories found there are, as far as we know, unparalleled in medieval Hebrew letters, and we shall give them our attention in this section as well. We must recall that we do not have the Arabic Vorlage from which he produced his translation, so we can only speculate what Arabic word lies behind the Hebrew. Indeed, as we have seen above, in our discussion of MSS Princeton and Tehran, there are numerous and significant differences even between versions of the same text. We will indicate in square brackets the passage where the term occurs, just as we did with regard to the Arabic terms.

Among the noteworthy medical terms are those used to render "warning", or "indication", as in the warning days that give notice that the crisis will soon be at hand: ימי הבְּשׂרָה, "warning days" [end of 13, 14], and מְבַשֵּׂר, "warning [day]" [18].[8] The second of these is paired with another unusual term, ימי המבט = "the days to be watched", i.e. the days on which the patient's condition should be observed closely; both are defined in [14]. Noteworthy as well are התאבקות, "disturbance" or "agitation" [1], and הבחראן השמור, "trustworthy crisis" [18], meaning a crisis that one can trust will not return. Finally, let us mention נֶעֱתַק, "relapsed" [3]; forms of this Hebrew verb are usually employed to translate forms of the Arabic *naqala*, with the general meaning of "movement" (including the movement from one language to another in the process of translation). In our text, the reasoning must be that a relapse is the movement of an illness from one period of time to another.

The interesting philosophy is found mainly at the beginning of Book

8 For a fuller discussion of the medical terms, see Gerrit Bos, *Novel Medical and General Hebrew Terminology from the 13th Century*. Vol. 2. *Journal of Semitic Studies*, Suppl. 30 (Oxford, 2013)

Three.[9] Shimshon ben Shlomo has not introduced any new words into the Hebrew philosophical lexicon; his terminology is well-attested. Herein, however, lies the true challenge: to choose the most appropriate English word for rather common terms, a selection that must be based upon the context and, to the extent possible, on the identification of the philosophical tradition to which the statement belongs. Consider this sentence: "That is to say, they [the Pythagoreans] thought it not be in vain that the worlds are three, i.e., the fixed world, the limited world, and the world that lies beneath the moon." [26] The Hebrew terms modifying the first two of the worlds are קיים and מוגבל. The second of these means is derived from the verb that means "to limit" and, by extension, "to define".[10] However, in the present context, מוגבל clearly means "limited", and it must correspond to πεπερασμένον, one of the terms used in the Pythagorean dichotomy limited—unlimited. The Hebrew term קיים, used to describe the first world, however, has a variety of meanings: "real", "existing", "fixed", "unmoving".[11] With some hesitation, we have chosen "unchanging"; see the notes to the passage. But in the following passage [27], the same word קיום appears together with העמדה, and there we have chosen to render the two terms "being" and "reality", as we explain in a note.[12]

The same passage [26] continues: "Rather, the reason for this is that the number three is primary, and so the worlds were divided up in this way." Again, the Hebrew מוקדם, which we have translated "primary" derives from a root (and an Arabic homonym), many forms of which are attested to, but its precise meaning in this context must be established.[13] The text immediately following clarifies: "and so the worlds were divided up in this way. For this very reason each of the species has one of the numbers especially [as-

9 The Arabic translation of Galen's *On Critical Days* is also very rich in this respect. Unfortunately, Cooper's translation and notes are particularly weak on those passages; see Y. Tzvi Langermann, "Critical Notes on a Study of Galen's *On Critical Days*, or A Study in Need of Critical Repairs," *Aestimatio* 9 (2012), 220-240.

10 See the numerous examples in Jacob Klatzkin, *Thesaurus Philosophicus Linguae Hebraicae* (New York, 1968), s.v. גבל; Klatzkin gives only one meaning, "definieren".

11 Klatzkin, s.v. קיים, gives two sets of meanings: "ruhend, unbeweglich" and "dauernd, dauerhaft, konstant". The second seems more appropriate here, especially in the sense used in Klatzkin's first example, drawn from a neoplatonic treatise by Isaac Israeli.

12 See further note 47 [page 97] to the translation below of the Hebrew version and Langermann, "The Astral connections of Critical Days", pp. 105-6.

13 See Klatzkin, 1:264, s.v. מקדם, who refers to it only in the sense of "cause" (סבה). An extensive discussion of the term features in Giuseppe Sermoneta, *Un glossario filosofico ebraico-italiano del XIII secolo* (Rome, 1969), no. 67.

sociated] with it." So it is because the number three, and number is general, is fundamental to reality that the worlds are a priori three, that crises recur on a given number of days, and so on. In this context, the best choice seems to be "primary", in the sense used, e.g., by Aristotle at the beginning of his Metaphysics (981b 29), when speaking of primary causes (πρῶτα αἴτια).

In [27], as we explain in a note, דמוי must mean representation [or: likeness], rather than "idea". שורש, "principle", literally "root", must be traced back eventually to the Greek ἀρχή.[14]

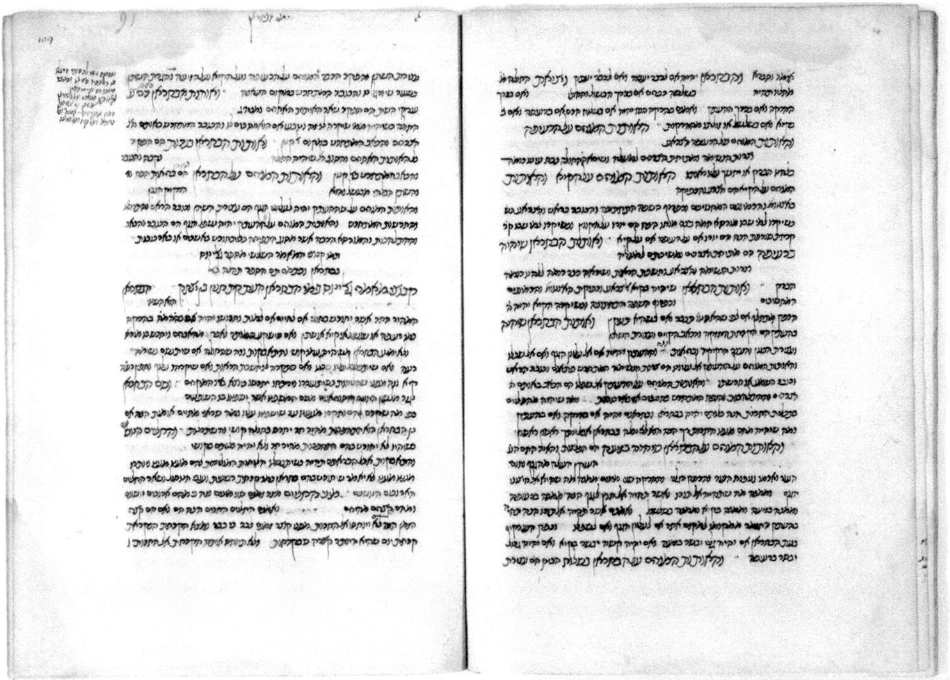

The Hebrew translation by Shimshon ben Shlomo features on fols. 104A-108b; it was copied in a Sephardic script in the 15th century; MS PARIS BIBLIOTHÈQUE NATIONALE DE FRANCE HÉB 1118, FOLS. 103B-104A.

14 Klatzkin, s.v. שרש, gives this term one of the longest entries in his lexicon (pp. 160-163 of part IV).

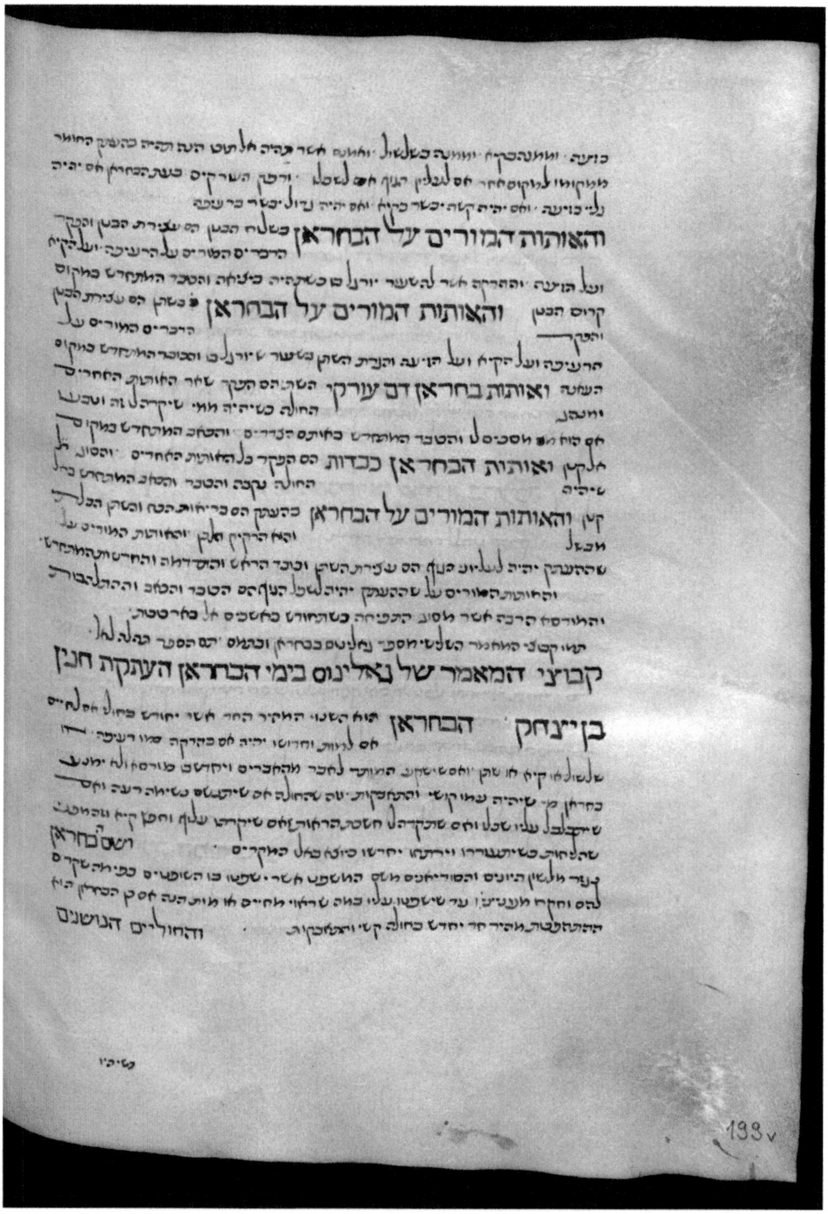

The Hebrew translation by Shimshon ben Shlomo features on fols. 199b-204a; it was copied in 1452 in a Sephardic script; MS VIENNA ÖSTERREICHISCHE NATIONALBIBLIOTHEK COD HEBR. 29 (CAT. SCHWARZ 174, 15), FOL. 199B.

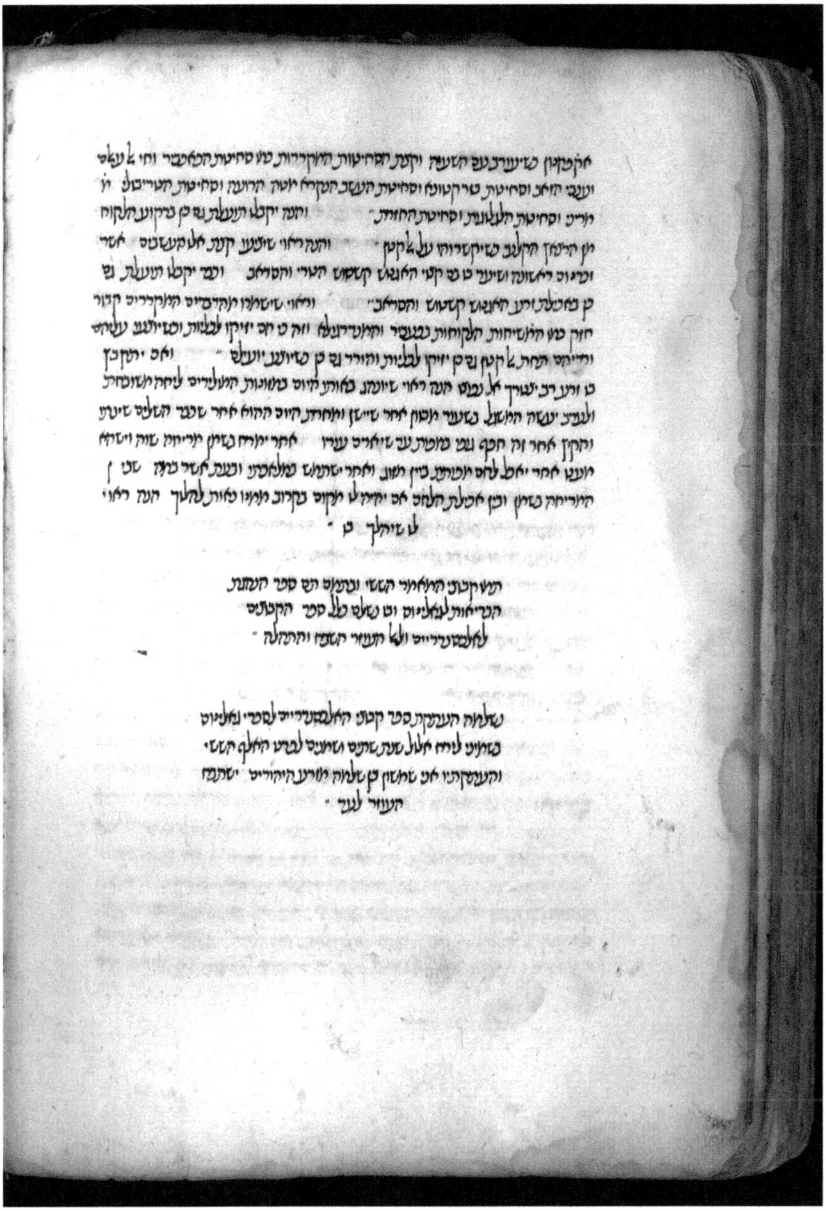

ST PETERSBURG, NATIONAL LIBRARY OF RUSSIA, HEBREW I 322, FOL 267V

The Hebrew Version

קבוצי מאמרי[1] גאלינוס בימי הבחראן העתקת חנין בן יצחק

[1] הבחראן הוא השנוי המהיר החד אשר יחודש בחולי אם לחיים אם למות וחדושו יהיה אם בהרקה כמו רעיפה או שלשול או קיא או שתן ואם שישקע המותר לאבר מהאברים ויחדש בו מורסא. ולא ימנע בחראן משיהיה[2] עמו קושי והתאבקות וזה שהחולה אם שיתנשם נשימה רעה ואם שיתבלבל עליו שכלו ואם שתקרה לו חשכת הראות ואם שיקרהו עלוף וחפץ קיא וזה מפני שהליחות כשיתעוררו וירתחו יחדשו כיוצא באלו המקרים. ושם הבחראן נגזר מלשון היונים והסוריאנים משם המשפט אשר ישפטו בו השופטים כפי מה שקדם להם וחקרו מענינו עד שישפטו עליו במה שראוי מחיים או מות הנה אם כן הבחראן הוא ההתהפכות מהיר חד יחדש בחולה קשי והתאבקות[3].

[2] והחוליים הנושנים כשיהיו לא יחודש בהם התהפכות מהיר[4] חד[5] ולא יהיה כלותם בקושי והתאבקות אבל הבראתם תהיה כשיתבשלו הליחות המולידות להם מעט מעט ויותכו[6] מעט מעט ולא יאמר שיחודש בהם בחראן כמו קדחת רביעית ועובי הטחול ושאר החוליים הארוכים הנושנים.

[3] מיני החוליים מצד זמנם שני מינים וזה כי מהם ארוכים נושנים[7] ומהם קצרים מהירים. ואמנם החוליים החדים הנה הם ואם הם קצרי הזמן הנה לא יוחסו אל החדות מפני קוצר זמנם לבד כי כבר נמצא הקדחת הנקראת קדחת יום שהיא היותר קצרה שבקדחות[8] ולא תיוחס אותה הקדחת אל החדות ולא יוחס מן החוליים אל החדות אלא מה שיתקבץ בו עם קוצר זמנו הסכנה. ואלו החוליים הם אשר יקראם אבוקראט חדים. והחוליים החדים מהם מה שיוחס[9] לתכלית החדות והם[10] אשר יבא[11] בהם[12] הבחראן בשביעי[13] או לפניו ומהם מיוחס לחדות על[14] השלוח והם אשר יבא הבחראן במה[15] שבין השביעי והי״ד. וכבר אמר אבוקראט שהחליים החדים יבא בהם הבחראן בארבעה עשר יום.

---

1 מאמרי: המאמר **אה**

2 משיהיה: מי שיהיה **אה**

3 והתאבקות: והשתכלות **ד**

4 מהיר: מה **אה**

5 חד: **אה** om

6 ויותכו מעט מעט: **א** om

7 נושנים: משנים **אה**

8 שבקדחות ולא תיוחס אותה הקדחת אל החדות ולא יוחס מן החוליים אל **ב**^{1}

9 שיוחס: שיינח **ג** אבוקראט **אה** add

10 והם: ואם **ג**

11 יבא: **ג**^{1} **ה** om

12 בהם הבחראן: **ה** inv

13 בשביעי:השביעי **א**

14 על: אל **ג**

15 במה שבין השביעי והי״ד: בארבעה עשר יום **אה** וכבר אמר אבוקראט שהחליים החדים יבא בהם הבחראן: **אה** om

ואמנם החליים שיארכו אחר ארבעה עשר עד שיגיעו אל הארבעים הנה יוחסו לחדות הנעתק לפי שהוא יחודש בו בימים הראשונים שיכלו בהם החוליים החדים בחראן חסר אחר לא יכלו כליון שלם במה שאחר זה מהימים עד הארבעים.

[4] ואמנם מה שיעבור זה מהחוליים הנה הוא יוחס כשהוא חולי ארוך ויוחס אל החדות למהירות תנועתו וזה שהחולי החד אמנם הוא החולי שיגיע תכליתו במהירות והפכו הוא המאוחר. ואם הנחנו שהבחראן אמנם הוא התהפכות המהיר החד[16] אשר עמו קושי והתאבקות הנה זה[17] ההתהפכות אמנם יהיה בחולי עד העשרים. ואמנם[18] מאחד ועשרים עד[19] הארבעים הנה כבר יהיה בחליים כליון מהיר חד תכוף אלא שהוא לא יהיה עמו קושי והתאבקות אבל יהיה ברוב העניינים בהעלם הראות או בשישקע המותר באבר מהאברים שיחדש בו מורסא. ואמנם אנחנו נקרא כליון החולי איך שיהיה בחראן ואם שיהיה בישולו מעט מעט והתוכו ההתוך שיעלם מהחוש וחוזק[20] הבחראן למספר השנים והחדשים. ועד יום העשרים הנה אמנם תהיה תנועת הבחראן בכל ארבעה ימים כמו שאמר אבוקראט.

[5] תנועת הבחראן וימי הבחראן. עוד כי תנועת[21] הבחראן וימי הבחראן יהיה אחר העשרים עד הארבעים בכל שבועות. עוד מאחר הארבעים תהיה תנועת הבחראן בכל[22] עשרים עד המאה ועשרים וימיו יעתקו אל מספר מהחדשים אחר אל[23] מספר מהשנים.

[6] והחליים שיחודש בהם הבחראן אמנם יודעו ממין החולי ר״ל מצורת החולי ומתנועתו. אמנם ממין[24] החולי ר״ל[25] צורתו הנה כמו הקדחת השורפת והקדחת השלישית שהם[26] ממיני החוליים שיבא הבחראן[27] בהם. ואמנם הקדחת הרביעית הנה ממיני החוליים שיבא בהם הבחראן מעט אבל כלותם יהיה מעט מעט. ואמנם תנועת החולי כי הוא כשיהיה מהיר ויהיה החם חזק יורה זה על חדוש הבחראן וכשתהיה תנועת החולי מאוחרת חלושה והחום בו מועט עוד לא[28] יחודש בו בחראן. ופעמים יהיה החולי מהחוליים שיחודש בהם בחראן ולא יבא בהם בחראן לחולשת הכח ולאותו מלדחות סבות החולי.

[7] וידיעת ימי הבחראן ממה שיצטרך לו הרופא בהקדמת הידיעה והבשורה עד שיקדים לחולה ויבשר במה שיהיה ויובטח בו בענייני החולים וירפאו על ידו כשירפאם במה שראוי ויקדים בהכנת[29] מה שיצטרך אליו קודם זמן הצורך לו וימלט שייוחס לו שהוא

---

16 החד: **ד** om
17 זה ההתהפכות אמנם יהיה בחולי עד העשרים: **ב¹**
18 ואמנם מאחד ועשרים: **ב** om
19 עד הארבעים הנה כבר יהיה בחליים כליון מהיר חד תכוף אלא שהוא לא יהיה עמו קושי והתאבקות **ב¹**
20 וחוזק: יחוזק **אבגה**
21 תנועת: תנועות **אה**
22 בכל: כל **ג**
23 אל: על **אה**
24 ממין: המין **אה**
25 ר״ל צורתו: **אה** om
26 שהם: **ד** om
27 הבחראן בהם: **ב** inv
28 לא: **ד** om
29 בהכנת מה: בהכית(?) במה **אה**

סיבת מות מי שימות.

[8] והבחראנים יבאו בזמן הגעת החוליים[30] ותכליתם אלא כשיקרה מקרה חזק ויכריח הטבע עד שיתעורר קודם העת הראוי מפני שהטבע אמנם יכון לדחיית[31] הליחות אחר שיבשלם וידקדקם וישיבם לעניין אשר יקל עמו הבדלם מהאברים.

[9] בשול החולי: ואמנם יורו[32] סבות החולי בעניין אשר ייוחס בהם אל שהם כבר נתבשלו כשהיו דביקות וסר מהם דבקותם[33] והיו עבות ודוקדקו או היו דקות[34] ונתעבו. וזה כלו אמנם יהיה וישלם בעת תכלית החולי ולזה הנה ראוי לרופא שיקדים וידע היום שיחודש בו הבחראן ויבוקש בו לחולה[35] המנוחה והמרגוע ולא יקריב לו ביום ההוא דבר מהרפואה ולא יניעהו בזולת זה תנועה חזקה רק יעזוב הטבע ישקוט וינוח עד שישלים פעלו והתאבקותו[36] לחולי ולא יטרידהו בחדוש יחדשהו[37] או דבר יקבלהו החולה.[38] וכבר אמר אבקראט שהוא מה שהתמיד החולי[39] בהתחלה הנה אם תראה להניעו[40] מעט הניעהו וכשהגיע החולי לתכליתו הנה עזיבת החולה[41] שוקט נח הוא יותר משובח.

[10] הנהגת המזון בעתות הבחראן[42] וידיעת ימי הבחראן: כבר יצטרך לה הרופא בהנהגת החולה והזנתו וזה שאין ראוי כשיקרב החולי[43] לתכליתו שיכביד הטבע המזון ויחלק[44] הטבע פעולתו ועסקו לטחינת המזון שיקח ולסיבות החולי. ולזה הנה ראוי אצל תכלית החולי שיעשה מההנהגה מה שהוא בתכלית הקצה מהדקות ושוה אמרך אצל תכלית החולי או שתאמר אצל סיבות החולי התם[45] הנשלם.

[11] ותכלית החולי מתחלף וזה שהוא כבר יהיה ביום הרביעי וכבר יתכן שתעשה מתחילת העניין ההנהגה אשר בתכלית הקצה מהדקות והוא שימנע[46] מהמאכל לגמרי וכשיהיה החולי תכליתו[47] מתאחר עד היום השביעי הנה בעליו יצטרך אל ההנהגה הדקה אשר לא תגיע בדקות[48] לתכליתו ויזון בתחילת העניין במי כשך השעורים או במי הדבש וכשיהיה תכלית החולי מתאחר עד יום הארבעה עשר הנה כבר יתכן שיזון בעליו בחלמון הביצה או במעט פתיתי הלחם הנקי. וכבר אמר אבוקראט כשיהיה חם חד יהיה חדוש

---

30 החוליים: החולים **אה**

31 לדחיית: לדחות **אה**

32 יורו: ילכו **אבדה**

33 דבקותם: דבקות **א** דבקו׳ **ה**

34 דקות: emendation editors דבקות MSS דקיקות **ד**[2]

35 לחולה: החולה **ג**

36 והתאבקותו: והתאבק **א** והתאבקות **גד**

37 יחדשהו: ויחדשהו **א**

38 החולה: החולי **ג**

39 החולי: החולה **אדה**

40 להניעו מעט: **ב** inv

41 החולה: החולי **ג**

42 הבחראן וידיעת ימי הבחראן: כבר יצטרך לה הרופא **ב**[1]

43 החולי: emendation editors החולה MSS

44 ויחלק: ויחלה **ב**

45 התם הנשלם: התכה נשלם **אה**

46 שימנע: **ב** om

47 תכליתו: לתכליתו **ד**

48 בדקות: בתכלית **אה**

הכאבים שהם בתכלית הקצה בו[49] נראים ויחוייב בהכרח שתעשה בו מההנהגה מה שהוא בתכלית הקצה מהדקות וכשלא יהיה כן איפשר בו ההנהגה שהיא יותר עבה. הנה כבר ראוי כפי רבות החולי ורחקו מהתכלית שתוסיף מעט במזון[50] וכשיגיע תכליתו ולפני זה מעט הנה[51] ראוי שיקל בו.

[12] הבחראן המשבח והבחראן המגונה: ואחר שיודע גבול התכלית ממין החולי ומתנועתו וזה שלא יעלם ממך החולי האם הוא מהחוליים המיוחסים אל החדות[52] יחס משולח ותנועת החולי איך היא במהירות ואיחור בלתי נאותה כשתפקוד תוספת החולי ותוספת הבשול בעת מעתות הבשורה[53] ומה שיקדם ויתחדש מהאותות קודם הבחראן הנה זה כבר יורה אותך על מהירותו ואיחורו. ואם היה כבר קדמו אותם האותות אותות משובחים[54] מורים על השלום ועל בישול החולי תדע שהבחראן יבא בטוב ובשלום ואם היה כבר קדמו אלה האותות אותות[55] רעים ולא קדמו אותות הבשול הנה זה אות[56] על שהבחראן יבא ברע.

[13] ואחר זה תדע שהידיעה[57] בדבר הבחראן ממה שכבר יצטרך לו[58] בהקדמת הידיעה במה שיהיה בהשערת המזון ובעשיית מה שיצטרך אליו מהידיעה בכל דבר ממנו בזמנו. וכמו שכבר יראו בעולם אותות תלקח הוראה בהם על מה שיהיה ויבשר בחדוש אותו הדבר המתחדש ויגביל זמן חדושו אם מהאותות שיראו בעולם ואם ממקומות הכוכבים כמו כן כבר יראו אותות מהטבע בשתן ודפק העורקים והיציאה ויורו על מה שיהיה מפעולת הטבע בהתאבקותו עם החולי האם הוא משובח או מגונה ויקראו אלו הימים שיראו בם אותם האותות ימי הבשורה וימי המבט.

[14] ימי הבשורה וימי המבט: וכמו שאין כל הימים ימי הבחראן כן אין כל הימים ימי בשורה אבל כאשר היה היום השביעי הוא יום הבחראן היה יום הרביעי הוא יום הבשורה בו עד שכשיראה בשתן ביום הרביעי ענן צף בעליונו או תלוי בו יהיה הבחראן בלי ספק ביום השביעי. וכל שבוע כשיחלק לשני חלקים הנה חלוקתו תפול ביום הרביעי והרביעי מכל שבוע יראה במה שיהיה ביום השביעי[59] ממנו לפי שהוא חולק השבוע לשני חלקים. וכמו כן הבחראן אם יבא כפי זה ביום הארבעה עשר היום[60] האחד עשר יבשר בו. ואל זה הענין כיון אבוקראט באמרו שחשבון ימי הבחראן יהיה על תוספת ארבעה[61] ארבעה עד העשרים. וכשיהפכו[62] ימי הבשורה[63] ויהיו ימי הבחראן יהיו אותם ההוראות

49 בו: **ד** om
50 במזון: מהמזון **ב**
51 הנה: זה מעט **אה** add
52 החדות: הסבות **ג**
53 הבשורה: **א** om
54 משובחים: משובחות **ב**
55 אותות: **א** om
56 אות: **ב** om
57 שהידיעה: **אה** om
58 לו: **ב** om
59 השביעי: השלישי **אה**^{2}
60 היום: הנה **אה**
61 ארבעה: **ב** om
62 וכשיהפכו: וכשיתהפכו **אה**
63 הבשורה: הבשורים **אה**

המבשרות בהם בימים אחרים מהימים אשר לפניהם. וכשיעברו ימי הבשורה העשרים תארך זמן בשורתם וזה שהם אמנם יבשרו בשבועות עד הארבעים.

[15] ואמנם יודעו ימי הבחראן ממה שכבר נשמר והובט פעמים רבות וזה שכל מה שהוא תחת עֹולם ההוייה וההפסד הנה שמושו יפול ברוב העִניינים במהלך הירח ולזה הנה ראוי שישפט עליו[64] במשפט ההכרחי. וכבר הובט ונשמר מימי הבחראן שהשביעי והארבעה עשר מהימים שיבא בהם היותר משבח שבבחראן ושהששי[65] מהימים שיבא בהם היותר רע שבבחראן ולא יהיה הבחראן בו אלא עם קשי והסתערות חזק. ופעמים יביא אל תוספת יהיה או אל מורסא תחודש בקצת האברים ולא ישובח מהבחראן מה שיפול בו בעליו בהתאבקות אחר וכשתהיה ביום הששי זיעה לא תהיה משתוה ולא בגוף כולו.

[16] העתק הבחראן ועברו גבולו והתאחרו מגבולו: והעתק הבחראן כשיקדים גבולו ויתאחר ממנו הוא לסבות רבות. הראשונה והיותר חזקה מהם שהסבות שיפלו תחת ההויה וההפסד ואפילו היו מתנועות[66] שמימיות הנה כבר נמצא הקף עתותיהם ויחוייב להם הסדור וישים מרוצת הטבע על הקפים אלא שאין אחד[67] מהם ממה שאי אפשר שיסור. אבל אמנם הוא מחוייב על הרב והסדור במה[68] שהוא נופל תחת ההוייה וההפסד אמנם הוא על הרב לא על עניין המחוייב בעניין אחד תמיד. וכבר איפשר שיתעורר הטבע לדחות מה שיזיקהו קודם העת המשבח לדחותו אם לרבויו אם לעקיצתו. ובכלל לחפיזה[69] תהיה מהסבה הפועלת כמו שההורג כבר יחפיזהו[70] קצת האברים[71] שיפילו המלחמה קודם העת שראוי בו הפלתו[72] לה. ואיפשר גם כן שיפשע החולה בנפשו ותהיה פשיעתו סבת העתק הבחראן מן זמנו. וכמו כן כבר איפשר שיהיה זה בפשיעה חדשה מי שחדשה לו או מהרופא הממונה ברפואתו או מהסבות שירדו עליו מחוץ כמו הבלגם והיגיעה והמחשבה והתעורה והפחד או מפני שנוי האויר. ולזה אמר אבוקראט אין ראוי לרופא שיסתפק על עשיית מה שראוי שיעשה מבלתי שיעזר[73] בחולה[74] על עצמו ובמי[75] שישמשהו ובאשר מחוץ.

[17] ופעמים ניחס[76] הבחראן אל יום בלתי יומו בסכלנו בזמן התחלת החולי שהוא הזמן שיפול בו החולה על המטה אבל התחלתו אמנם היא התחלת לקיחת הקדחת. והרבה מהאנשים יקרה להם החולי ויכריחום[77] עניינים בעת ההוא עד שיתעסקו במה שהיה

---

64 עליו: לא **אבגד** add

65 ושהששי: שיבא **אה** add ושהששי מהימים שיבא בהם היותר רע: **ד** om ושהששי מהימים שיבוא בהם היותר רע **ד**^{1}

66 מתנועות: מתנועעות **אה**

67 אחד: **אה** om

68 במה: שיצא **א** add

69 לחפיזה: לזפזה(!) **אה** לחפזה **בד**

70 יחפיזהו: יחפיהו(!) **אה** יחפזהו **בד**

71 האברים: הדברים **בד**

72 הפלתו: הפלגתו **ב**

73 שיעזר: **אה** om

74 בחולה: emendation editors בחולי **אגדה**

75 ובמי שישמשהו: emendation editors ובמי שימששהו **גד** וכמו שימשכהו **אה** שישמשהו **ד**^{2}

76 ניחס: כיחס **אה**

77 ויכריחום: נכריחום **אה**

מנהגם להשתמש בו[78] בעת הבריאות. ופעמים ילאה הטבע גם כן מלדחות החולי בכללו ביום אחד עד שיצטרך להתאחר עד יום אחר ויוחס הבחראן אל היום השני כמו מה שיהיה הבחראן ביום השביעי ולא יתחזק הטבע על דחיית החולי בכללו באותו היום ויצטרך בדחיתו למה שישאר ממנו אל היום השמיני ויוחס הבחראן בסבת זה אל השמיני. ופעמים יהיו לקדחת גם כן הקיפים באים בזוגות כמו שיקרה בשלישית הכפולה. ויהיה ממנהג[79] החולי שיבא בו הבחראן בשביעי או בתשיעי ויפול בשמיני או בששי קושי הקדחת ועצרה הטבע מלפתוח לדחות[80] מה שכבר הוכן לדחותו ואעפ״י שלא היתה הכנתו נשלמת. לאלו הסבות כולם כבר יפול הבחראן בזולת ימיו ויפסד גבול יום הבחראן האמיתי.

[18] הבחראן השלם והבחראן החסר: וכבר ראוי שיתקבץ בבחראן שיהיה שלם ושיהיה שמור ושיהיה[81] ביום הבחראן בטוח ושיהיה מבואר ואשר לו מבשר והבחראן הרע המגונה הוא מה שיהיה לו הפכי אלו העניינים. והבחראן השלם הוא הבחראן שיותך בו החולי כלו עד שלא ישאר בגוף מסבותיו דבר. והבחראן השמור הוא הבחראן שיובטח עמו שהחולי לא ישוב. וכבר יאמר לזה בעצמו בחראן אמיתי ובחראן בטוח ורחוק מהסכנה. ואמנם יהיה הבחראן שמור כשקדמוהו אותות הבשול והיה חדושם ביום מימי הבחראן שיובטח בהם. והבחראן הבטוח הוא הבחראן שלא[82] יהיו עמו מקרים בהם סכנה כמו הדפיקה וכאב הקרבים וזולת זה ממה שדומה להם. והבחראן המבואר הוא אשר סבות כלות החולי בו מבוארות גלויות כמו הזיעה והשלשול ודומיהם. והבחראן המבושר בו הוא הבחראן שקדמוהו אותותיו ביום מימי הבשורה וזה שהטבע לא יגש אל החוליים פתאם אבל אמנם יעשה בהם מעט מעט עד שינצחם הנה הוא כשילך[83] בו ידחם בימי הבשורה. עתה יזכור התחלף ימי הבחראן.

[19] המאמר השני ימי הבחראן והדרגתם: מימי הבחראן ימים הם היותר חזקים והיותר משובחים והם היום השביעי והיום הארבעה עשר כי אלו הימים מימי הבחראן הם המשבחים מימי הבחראן שבין התחלת החולי ליום העשרים ממנו והיותר בטוחים. עוד הימים השניים אחר אלו הימים המבשרים בהם והם הרביעי והאחד עשר והשבעה עשר. עוד השלישיים אחר אלו הם הימים שבמה שבין אלו שיתקדם בהם הבחראן או יתאחר. אמנם מהיום הרביעי הנה הם היום השלישי והיום החמישי ואמנם מהיום השביעי הנה הם היום הששי והיום השמיני. ואמנם הבחראן שיהיה ביום האחד עשר הנה רב מה שיתקדם הוא ביום התשיעי בחפזת[84] כח הקדחת. ואלו הם הימים שיחדש בהם הבחראן המשבח ברוב העניינים. ומהם היום הששי והיום הזה כאילו ימשך היום השביעי כחו וימשול עליו אבל הוא לא יהיה בו הבחראן על דרך השלום ולא על דרך שלמות וזה שלא

---

78 בו: **ד** om

79 ממנהג: מהמנהג **אה**

80 לדחות: לחות **אה**

81 ושיהיה: ובשיהיה **אה** ושיהיה ביום הבחראן בטוח: ויהיה בטוח ביום הבחראן **ג**

82 שלא יהיו: שיהיו **ד**

83 כשילך: בשולך(?) **ג**

84 בחפזת: בחכזת **ג**

תשתלח בו[85] זיעה נגרת משתוה ולא ישוב כבחראן שיהיה בו הכח[86] השביעי[87] אצלך כאשר הנהיג עניינו במדרגת המלך הטוב ומדרגת היום הששי במדרגת המתגבר הרע. ואי אפשר לבחראן ההווה בעשרים שיבא בהם האחד ועשרים יום[88] אלא בבשורה ועם זה יהיה היום המבשר בו היום השמונה עשר. ואמנם היום השלשה עשר הנה הוא חלוף הימים שיחודש בהם הבחראן לגמרי בעניין מהעניינים לפי שהוא חסר הכח מכל ימי הבחראן. ואמנם היום השני הנה לא יחודש בו הבחראן בעניין מן העניינים מפני שהכח עדיין חזק ויסבול מה שיזיקהו עד שלא יתעורר קודם העת שראוי שיתעורר בו.

[20] הימים אשר אין בהם הבחראן ולא יחודש[89] הבחראן[90] ג״כ בעניין מהעניינים ביום החמשה עשר ולא ביום הששה עשר ולא ביום התשעה עשר לפי שיום[91] החמשה עשר שני ליום הארבעה עשר ויום הששה עשר יתקדם ליום השבעה עשר ויום[92] התשעה עשר מתקדם ליום העשרים. והשבועות שיחודש בהם[93] הבחראן מהם שיחשבו על הדבקות ומהם שיחשבו על ההפרדה.

[21] הפרדת השבועות והקף הארבעה[94] המבשרים: ואמנם המשבח מהם על ההפרדה הנה השבוע הראשון והשבוע השני ואמנם המשבח מהם על הדבקות הנה בשבוע השני והשבוע השלישי וזה שיום הבחראן כפי חשבון ימי השבועות מיום הארבעה עשר איננו יום האחד ועשרים אבל הוא יום העשרים מפני שיום הארבעה עשר הוא התחלת השבוע השלישי. והימים ג״כ שיחשבו על הקף הארבעה המבשרים בבחראן המתחדשת בשבועות אמנם ינהג חשבונם מנהג חשבון השבועות. והיותר עצום מה שיהיה מההתאבקות והקושי מהבחראן אשר יהיה עד[95] יום הארבעה עשר והבחראן מזה העת יהיה בו מן הקושי וההתאבקות. וכמו כן גם כן הנה ימי הבחראן הנופלים בין ימיהם המתחדשים על חשבון הסבובים[96] ולא יפול אחר הארבעה עשר עוד אחר העשרים הנה ימי הבשורה שיהיו על חשבון הארבעה עשר[97] הנה הם יחלשו. וזה שהבשורה אמנם תהיה אצל זה[98] בשבועות וסבובי השבועות גם כן מאחר יום הארבעים יחלשו וזה שהתנועה אמנם תהיה אצל זה בכל עשרים עד שיהיה הבחראן ביום הארבעים עוד ביום הששים עוד ביום השמונים עוד ביום המאה עוד ביום המאה ועשרים עוד יתאחר אחר כן הבחראן ויהיה בהמשכות המניין.

[22] וכבר אמר אבוקראט שהחולים הקיציים יותכו בסתו והחליים הסתוים יותכו בקיץ. וכבר זכר מהבחראן מה שיהיה מהסבובים יותר רחוק מאלו ואמר שהרבה מהחוליים בנ־

---

85 בו: **ד** om

86 הכח: עד שיהיה **ד** add עד שיהיה במדרגת **ב** add במדרגת **ד**^{1} add

87 השביעי אצלך כאשר הנהיג עניינו: **ד**^{1}

88 יום: **ד** om

89 יחודש: **אה** ditt

90 הבחראן: **אה** om

91 שיום: שביום **ד**

92 ויום התשעה עשר: **בד** om והתשעה עשר **ד**^{1}

93 בהם: ביום **אה**

94 הארבעה: **אה** om

95 עד: על **אה**

96 הסבובים: ההבובים(!) **אה**

97 עשר: **אגדה** om

98 זה: **ד**^{2}

ערים מהם מה שיכלו[99] חלק בע׳[100] ומהם מה שיכלו בשבעה חדשים ומהם בשבעה שנים ומהם כשיקרבו לצמיחת השער בגב הערוה. ואמנם[101] אבוקראט בספר אפידימיא לפי שהיה[102] הספר הזה אמנם שמו מזכרת[103] לו זכר כל הימים שיחודש בהם הבחראן ר״ל הימים שייחד טבעם הבחראן והימים אשר יטו בכח הבחראן על היום שהוא ראשון בו.

[23] ואמנם בספר הפרקים ובספר הקדמת הידיעה הנה אמנם זכר הימים שיחודש בהם הבחראן על[104] שהוא מיוחד בטבעם וממה שזכרו מימי הבחראן במאמר הראשון מספר אפידימיא אמנם מהזוגיים הנה הרביעי והששי והשמיני והארבעה עשר והשמונה עשר והארבעה ושלשים והארבעים והששים והשמונים והמאה והמאה ועשרים. ואמנם מהנפרדים הנה השלישי והחמשי והשביעי והתשיעי והאחד עשר והשבעה עשר והאחד ועשרים והאחד ושלשים. ואמנם בספר הפרקים ובספר הקדמת הידיעה הנה חייב הבחראן לשביעיות ולרביעיות ואמר[105] בספר הפרקים שהחליים החדים יבא בהם הבחראן בארבעה עשר יום ושהמבשר ביום השביעי הוא היום הרביעי והיום השמיני הוא התחלת שבוע אחר ושהיום המבשר אחר זה הוא האחד עשר וזה שהיום הזה הוא[106] היום המבשר בשבוע האחר. עוד המבשר בשבוע השלישי אחר כן הוא היום[107] השבעה עשר לפי שזה הוא רביעי ליום הארבעה עשר ושביעי לאחד עשר.

[24] ואמנם בספר הקדמת הידיעה אמר שהקדחות יכלו במספרים[108] בעצמם מהימים בהם ישלם מי שישלם ויאבד מי שיאבד. וזה שהיותר שלמה שבקדחות והיותר בטוחת[109] האותות תשקוט ביום הרביעי או לפניו והיותר[110] קשה שבקדחות והיותר רעת[111] האותות תמית[112] ביום הרביעי או לפניו. ועד כה יגיע סבובם הראשון.[113] ואמנם סבובם השני הנה יכלה אל השביעי ואמנם סבובם השלישי הנה יכלה ליום האחד עשר ואמנם סבובם הרביעי הנה יכלה ליום הארבעה עשר ואמנם סיבובם החמישי הנה יכלה ליום השבעה עשר ואמנם סבובם הששי הנה יכלה ליום העשרים. ואלו הסבובים על התוספת יגיעו עד יום העשרים ואי איפשר שיחשב דבר מזה על חשבון ימים שלמים מפני[114] שהשנה גם כן והחדשים[115] לא יתכן שיחשבו על חשבון ימים שלמים. עוד כפי זאת

99 שיכלו: שיוכלו **ב**
100 בע׳: **אבדה** om
101 ואמנם: ואמר **גד**
102 שהיה: שיהיה **אה**
103 מזכרת: מוכרת **א**
104 על שהוא מיוחד בטבעם וממה שזכרו מימי הבחראן: **אה** om
105 ואמר: ואמנם **אגה**
106 הוא: **ד** om
107 היום: **אה** om
108 במספרים: במספרי העונות **אה**
109 בטוחת: בטוחות **אבדה**
110 והיותר קשה שבקדחות והיותר רעת האותות תמית ביום הרביעי או לפניו: **ד**¹
111 רעת: בטוחת אה רעת **ה**¹
112 תמית: תמות **אבה**
113 הראשון: **ב**¹
114 מפני שהשנה גם כן והחדשים לא יתכן שיחשבו על חשבון ימים שלמים: **אה** om
115 והחדשים: גם כן **ב** add

ההנהגה מהתוספת יהיה הסבוב הראשון יום[116] הארבעה ושלשים. עוד[117] הסבוב השני יום הארבעים עוד הסבוב השלישי יום הששים.

[25] ואמר שהעלה בשבוע השלישי כפי עלות הדבקות שהחודש לא ירוץ חשבונו על ימים שלימים תמימים. וזה שהיותר גדול שבשרשים הטבעיים[118] שמה שבשמים יפעֵל מה שבארץ ובייחוד הירח להיותו היותר קרוב ממה שבשמים לארץ. והעתק הירח יהיה לא בסבובו שיתחבר[119] בו עם השמש שיהיה בקרוב מתשעה ועשרים אבל בסבובו בגלגל המזלות שיהיה בשבעה ועשרים יום ושליש. וכאשר חלקו אלו הימים לארבעה רבועים[120] לפי שרבועי הירח כשיוקשו בהקש גלגל המזלות יותר חזק ולא יתחלקו בהקש סבוב הירח עד שיגיע לשמש יהיה רבוע הירח ששה ימים וחצי ושליש יום. ולזה יכלה השבוע השלישי ביום העשרים ולא יכלה ביום האחד ועשרים והשבוע השני יכלה ליום הארבעה עשר. ואמנם ימנה יום[121] העשרים בבחראן לפי שחציו יתחיל בו[122] יום[123] אחרון מהשבוע השלישי וילחם הבחראן עד חציו. עתה יזכור עלות ימי הבחראן.

[26] המאמר השלישי: אמר שפיתאגורש וסיעתו יחסו העלות של ימי הבחראן אל המספרים. וחייבו למה שיסוב בשמים מהכוכבים פעולות במה שילוה להם מהתחלף תמונותיהם וחייבו עם זה למספר אשר אחר סבובי מה שיחודש כמה שבארנו כח יחודש עונות עתים במה שיחודשו. ויהיה זה שהם חשבו[124] שלא היו לבטלה העולמות השלשה ר״ל העולם הקיים והעולם המוגבל והעולם אשר למטה מהירח אבל אמנם היה זה מפני שמספר השלשה היה מוקדם ונחלקו העולמות על זאת החלוקה. ולזאת הסבה היה מיוחד כל אחד מהמינים אחד מהמספרים ואם לא מה עניין הדבר בחוליים[125] החדים[126] שיכלו ברביעיות והשביעיות והחוליים[127] הנושנים יכלו בכל עשרים יום לולי שמה שיחויב[128] בגלגל כבר[129] יחויב[130] במה שירוץ על זולת מנהג הטבע[131] כ״ש מבלתי שעורים מתחלפים. ולזה[132] היה היום הששי והיום השמיני והם יחד[133] יפלו על קדחת ביותר רע שבבחראן.

[27] ואמנם גאלינוס הנה הדבר אצלו אל המספר אמנם הוא דמוי יחשבהו האדם במחש־

---

116 יום: נ״א יום השני<ם> ועשרים נ״א שהעשרים **ד**[1]

117 עוד: **א** om עו׳ **ה**

118 הטבעיים שמה שבשמים: **אה** om

119 שיתחבר: **א** om

120 רבועים: רביעיים **ב**

121 יום: **אה** om

122 בו: ביום **אה**

123 יום: ליום ו עשרים <...>ה פעמי׳ <...>צי ושליש <...> וחצי העשרים <הא>חרון **ד**[1] add

124 חשבו: יחשבו **אה**[1]

125 בחוליים: בחולים **אה**

126 החדים: **אה** om

127 והחוליים: והחולנים **אה**

128 שיחויב: שיסוב **אבה**

129 כבר: דבר **אבה**

130 יחויב יחייב **אבה**

131 הטבע: הטבעי **א**

132 ולזה: כך פריס 884 ולמה אבדה <...> **ג**

133 יחד: נ״א קרובים **ד**[2]

בה ואיננו אצלו ממה שלו העמדה וקיום ומציאות שורש ולזה נאץ מאמרים רבים מחברי ארסטו׳ המיוחסים אל המשאים ואמר שהוא שוה אם אמר האומר שהיום השביעי הוא

[28] יום בחראן או[134] ששערי המדינות[135] אל המדינת אסא שבעה מאמרים. אמנם היה[136] היום השביעי יום בחראן במקום[137] מספר השבעה ולא יחבר עניין כל הבחראן אלא אל תמונות[138] הירח ויחשוב ששאר הכוכבים כבר יפעלו עליותיהם ותמונותיהם פעלות בנו ולא יהיו פעולותיהם בעניינים הכוללים מחדושי הקיץ והסתו אבל כבר יהיו פעולותיהם בעניינים המיוחדים. ואמנם הירח הנה פעולותיו שני מינים אחד מהם במהלכו עד שישוב אל השמש והאחר במהלכו בעגלתו[139] בגלגל המזלות ואמנם[140] סבוב הירח עד שישיג השמש וזה[141] הסבוב יהיה[142] בתשעה ועשרים יום וחצי.[143] ואמנם[144] העת שיסוב בו הירח בעגלתו בגלגל המזלות הנה יהיה משבעה ועשרים יום ושליש. ואמ׳ שתמונות הירח בהקשו אל השמש יחדשו פעולות כוללות. ואמנם תמונותיו בהקש עגלתו בגלגל המזלות הנה יחדשו[145] פעולות[146] הם יותר מיוחדות מאותם ושהיותר חזק שבתמונות הירח התמונות שיהיו חצי עגלה והם התמונות שיהיה בהם מהשמש על תכלית הרחק. עוד אחריהם התמונות שיהיה[147] בהם הירח בעל שני גבולים ושהחלושה[148] שבתמונות שתהיה בהם הירח תמונתו בראשית עלייתו ושהתחלת סבוב הירח בהקש[149] סבובו בגלגלהמזלות[150] היום שהתחיל בו החולי בחולה וכפי הקש זה היום ראוי שיובטו ויחשבו הסבובים.

[29] ואמנם מאמר גאלינוס שהימים השלשה שיעלם בהם הירח לא יפעל בהם הירח פעלה בארץ ולזה יתחבר על[151] העניין היותר קרוב מהלך הירח עד שישיג השמש במהלכו בגלגלו בגלגל המזלות הנה אנחנו לא נקבלהו ממנו וזה שלא יחוייב מפני שאצל הסתר הירח לא ינשבו הרוחות ואמנם ינשבו עם הגלותו.

[30] הירח פעולתו בארץ: אבל כבר ראוי לנו שנקבל ממנו מה שאמרו והטיב באמרו שפעולות הירח בחשבון החולי אמנם יהיו על הקש סבובו בגלגל המזלות אבל שהוא מתחלף כפי תמונותיו בהקש השמש וזה שרבוע הירח כבר יפעל לא בהקש החולי לבד אבל

---

134 או: emendation editors אלא MSS נ״א אל **ד**[2]
135 המדינות אל המדינת אסא שבעה מאמרים: إنّ مدينة ثبين سبعة أبواب CG 377, l. 10
136 היה: **אה** om
137 במקום: למקום **אה**
138 תמונות: תמונת **אה**
139 בעגלתו: פעולתו **א** בעגלתו **א**[1]
140 ואמנם: והוא **בא**[1]
141 וזה: הנה זה **אה**
142 יהיה: היה **אבה**
143 וחצי: ושליש **ד**
144 ואמנם העת שיסוב בו הירח בעגלתו בגלגל המזלות הנה יהיה משבעה ועשרים יום: **ב** om
145 יחדשו: יחודש **אה**
146 פעולות הם: פעולותיהם **אה**
147 שיהיה: חצי עגלה **אה** add
148 ושהחלושה: ושהחולשה **א**
149 בהקש: בהקשו **אה**
150 המזלות: הנה יחודשו פעולותיהם יותר מיוחדות מאותם ושהיותר חזק שבתמונות הירח התמונות **אה** add
151 על: **אה** om

כבר הוא יפעל בהקש השמש. וכמו כן התמונות בהקש שאר הכוכבים והעתקתם[152]
ג״ב כשיגיע[153] לתכלית[154] בחולי מהחוליים נמצא בזה התהפכות מעניין לעניין. וכמו
[31] כן עליית הכוכבים המפורסמים ושקיעתם. וכפי זה אמר אבוקראט ששתיית הרפואה
קודם עֲליית[155] אל שערי אל עבור ואחר עלייתו קשה. ואין ראוי שיושמו עליות הכוכבים
ושקיעותיהם אותות לעתות השנה ומה שיחודש בהם לבד אחר שכבר יפעלו פעולות
במה שאין נפש לו. ומזה שהשמש כבר יתהפך בעת התהפכו בזמן ההתהפכות[156] הקיצי
והימים כמו שאמ׳ באוקרסטאס לא יהיו[157] אדומיים[158] מעלית אל סמאך אל רמאח
מפני שבעלייתו כח בורר להם. ואמנם השינויים שיהיו כפי החדשים הנה אמנם יחודשו
עם הירח כאשר יורה מה שבים מהב״ח ובפרט[159] הבעל חיים המכסה חרסים וזה שזה
הב״ח יתנועע בתנועת הירח ויתוסף עמו ויחסר[160] עמו. והכפייה ג״ב אמנם יהיה הת־
עוררותה כפי חשבון החדש בזמן התחסרו ורחק הירח במה[161] שיהיה כפי חשבון הקש
החדש יהיו הרוחות שיחודשו[162] בעת עליית הירח משתנות[163] אצל היות הירח חצי
עגלה. והרוחות שיחודשו[164] אצל היות הירח חצי עגלה ישתנו אצל שלמותו והרוחות
[32] שיחודשו[165] אצל שלמות הירח ישתנו אצל היותו שנית חצי עגלה. וככה אמר ארסטו.[166]
הנה כבר התבאר שראוי שיחוייב גדול[167] הכח ליום השביעי וליום[168] הארבעה עשר
אחר שהרבוע[169] והנגוד אמנם יהיו בשתי אלו התמונות. ואמנם התמונה שיהיה עליה
הירח בראשית עלייתו הנה עמידה תהיה ברביעי וכמו כן התמונה שהיא בעלת שני גבו־
לים והיא[170] על השלוש[171] תשמש[172] אל האחד עשר. והשמש לפי שהוא פועל בהוייה
יהיו שנוייו בגבולים שהם יותר גדולים.[173] תמו קבוצי המאמר השלישי מספר ימי[174]
הבחראן לגאלינוס ובתמם תם הספר ת״ל.

---

152 והעתקתם: והעתקתים **אה**
153 כשיגיע: כשיגיעו **א**
154 לתכלית: בתכלית **אה**
155 עליית: **אה** om
156 ההתהפכות: התהפכות **אה**
157 יהיו: היו **אה**
158 אדומיים: אדמים **אה**
159 ובפרט הבעל חיים: **אה** om
160 ויחסר עמו: **אה** om
161 במה: למה **אה**
162 שיחודשו: שיחודש **אה**
163 משתנות: **אה** om
164 שיחודשו: יחודשו **אה**
165 שיחודשו: **א** om יחודשו **ה**
166 ארסטו: אראטס **אה**
167 גדול: גודל **אה**
168 וליום: וביום **א**
169 שהרבוע: הרבוע **אה**
170 והיא: והוא **ב**
171 השלוש: השליש **אה**
172 תשמש: תשמר **אה**
173 גדולים: גבולים **א**
174 ימי: **ד** om

CHAPTER 6

The Translation of the Hebrew Version

The [Hebrew] Summaries of Galen's books[1] *On Critical Days*, from the [Arabic] by Ḥunayn ibn Isḥāq

[1] A crisis is a swift, sudden change that occurs in an illness, either for life or for death.[2] It occurs either through evacuation, such as a nosebleed or diarrhea or emesis or urine, or through a residue that settles in an organ and causes an inflammation. A crisis is unavoidably accompanied by hardness and struggle, namely that the patient has breathing problems, or that he is delirious, suffers from dimsightedness, fainting, or nausea. For when humors are stirred up and [begin to] boil they cause symptoms of that sort. The term "BHR'N" [i.e., Arab. *buḥrān*] is derived from Greek[3] and Syriac[4] [in which it means] the verdict of life or death made by the judges on the basis of their preceeding investigation.[5] Thus, a crisis is a fast, sudden change, which causes hardness and struggle to the patient.

[2] Chronic illnesses do not have a fast, sudden change and do not end with hardness and struggle, but they are cured when the humours that cause [these illnesses] become concocted and dissolve little by little, and [so] it cannot be said that a crisis happens to them. Examples [of such illnesses] are quartan fever, thickness of the spleen and all the prolonged, chronic illnesses.

[3] There are two kinds of illnesses with regard to their length, namely

---

1 I.e., the three books that make up his treatise *On Critical Days*.

2 Cf. Langermann, "Astral Connections", p. 103: "The crisis of a fever is a swift change in its development"; cf. Galen, *In Hippocratis Aphorismos Commentarius II* (K 17b.470): Ἡ μὲν κρίσις ὀξυρροπός ἐστιν ἐν νόσῳ μεταβολὴ πρὸς ὑγειάν ἢ θάνατον (A crisis is a sudden and swift change in a disease either for health or for death).

3 I.e.. κρίσις; cf. H.G. Liddell and R. Scott, *A Greek English Lexicon* (repr. Oxford 1989), p. 997: "separating, distinguishing; 2. decision, judgement..., II. judgement of a court..."

4 I.e., *Buḥrānā*; cf. C. Brockelmann, *Lexicon Syriacum* (Halle 1928), p. 65: "1. examinatio; 2. crisis (morbi)." Cf. the marginal note in Galen, *Buḥrān*, MS London, fol. 59r: *al-buḥrānu ismun Suryāniyyun wa-maʿnāhu l-ḥukmu.*

5 At the beginning of the third part of *On Critical Days* (K 9.704,17705,5), Galen explains the etymology of this term. According to him, it was not a physician who called this stage of a disease for the first time "judgement." The inventor of this term was rather a layman, who saw a sick person in the state of a crisis. Frightened by this terrible sight, he compared the state of this patient to that of someone being on trial for murder and waiting for judgment.

 | DOI 10.1163/9789004282223_007

those that are prolonged and chronic and those that are short and fast. Acute illnesses, although they are short, are not considered to be acute only because of their shortness, for [there are illnesses] like ephemeral fever which is the shortest of the fevers but is not considered to be acute. Illnesses are considered to be acute only when shortness is combined with danger. These are the illnesses which Hippocrates calls "acute". Of[6] the acute illnesses there are those that are considered to be extremely acute, namely those in which the crisis occurs on or before the seventh day, and there are those which are considered to be acute in a general sense,[7] namely those in which the crisis comes between the seventh and fourteenth day. Hippocrates[8] has said that in acute illnesses the crisis comes on the fourteenth day. In the case of illnesses that last after the fourteenth day, they are considered to be acute from[9] the relapse, until they reach the fortieth day, since[10] a defective crisis happens in them in the first days during which acute illnesses resolve, and since their resolution will not be complete in the following days until the fortieth.

[4] Illnesses that are prolonged beyond this [day fourteen] will be considered to be long-lasting, but they will be considered to be acute on account of their swift movement; for an acute illness is that illness whose end comes fast while it is slow when the opposite is the case. If we have assumed that a crisis is a fast, acute change which is accompanied by hardness and agitation, then this change occurs in an illness up to the twentieth [day]. From the twenty-first until the fortieth day illnesses have a fast, acute, immediate

---

6 Cf. Ḥunayn, trans. Cooper, CG 298-9 (=K 886.11): "So let us call the illnesses that linger to the seventh day 'very acute'".

7 Hebrew על השלוח or משולח (see [12] below), corresponding to Arabic مرسل, means in a general, non-specific sense.

8 Cf. Hippocrates, *Aphorisms* 2.23 (Loeb Classical Library, London 1931, repr. 1979), p. 113: "Acute diseases come to a crisis in fourteen days"; cf. idem, *Crises* 14 (Loeb Classical Library, London 2010), p. 283: "Acute diseases have their crises in fourteen days in most cases"; see as well CG 288-289 (K 880.11).

9 "acute from the relapse" (מן הנעתק): cf. Ḥunayn, CG 301, l.1 (K 887.1): حادّا عارضا من التنكّس (from the relapse, trans. Cooper), ibid. note 897: acute from the relapse: μέχρι τῆς τεσσαρακοστῆς add K ("up to the fourteeth day"). It is called this because if the illness has lasted that long, it *must* have relapsed at least once by then.

10 "since a defective crisis happens in them in the first days during which acute illnesses resolve"; cf. CG, p. 300 (K. 887.2): "the first days during which acute illnesses resolve and since their resolution will not be complete in the following days until the fourteeth"; cf. CG 300-1 (K 887.2-4): "which must be called by this name only when there is a defective crisis in an acute illness in the twentieth day or before it, the strength of its remaining part is broken (and) its resolution will occur in the fortieth day or before".

end, but it does not come with hardness and agitation, as it comes in most cases while it is hidden from the eye or when a residue settles in an organ in which it causes an inflammation. But we call the end of the disease, however it may be (i.e. clear agitation or some other bodily event) a crisis, even if its concoction is slow and its dissolution is such that it is hidden from the senses. The strength of the crisis is [in keeping with?] the years and months. Up to[11] the twentieth day the motion of the crisis is every four days as Hippocrates said.

[5] The motion of the crisis and the days of the crisis: The motion of the crisis and the days of the crisis after the twentieth until the fortieth are [reckoned] according to weeks. After[12] forty [days] the motion of the crisis is [reckoned] every twenty [days] until one hundred and twenty [days] and [then] its [critical] days are transferred to the number of months and then to the number of years.

[6] The diseases in which a crisis occurs are known according to the kind of disease; that is, its form and its motion. As for [knowing it from the] kind of illness, i.e. its form, it is like ardent fever and tertian fever, for these are the kinds of diseases that have a crisis. But quartan fever belongs to the kinds of diseases that only have a minor crisis and that have a slow resolution. If the motion of the illness is fast and the fever strong, it indicates the occurrence of a crisis. And if the motion of the illness is slow [and] weak and the fever is minor, a crisis does not yet happen in it. Sometimes an illness is one of those illnesses in which a crisis can happen, but it does not [actually] happen because of the weakness of the power [of the body] and its inability to repel the causes of the illness.

[7] The knowledge of the days of the crisis is part of what a physician needs for a prognosis and warning[13] so that he can warn the patient beforehand about what will happen. Thus, he will be trustworthy in the matters that concern patients. They will be cured by him, as he will give them a proper treatment and prepare beforehand what he needs subsequently. He will not then be held responsible when a patient dies.

[8] Crises happen when illnesses reach a climax unless a serious accident occurs which forces nature to become active before the proper time,

---

11 Cf. Hippocrates, *Crises* 7, p. 279: "that is, these increments in the most acute (sc. of fevers) are by fours up to the number twenty". See also CG 290-291 (K 881.15-17), on the three types of illness: those whose crisis occurs in days, those whose crisis occurs in months, and those whose crisis occurs in years.

12 Cf. CG 182-3 (K 817.9-11): "It is my view that Hippocrates disparaged all of the days after the fortieth day, except for the sixtieth, the eightieth, and the hundred-twentieth day."

13 "warning" (בשורה); cf. below section 14.

because nature strives to expel the residues once they have been concocted, dissolved, and reduced to a state in which their expulsion from the organs is easy.

[9] The concoction of an illness: An indication for the [humoural] causes of an illness to be considered as concocted is when they are viscous or not viscous anymore, or that they were thick and then became fine, or that they were fine and then turned thick. All this will be complete at the time of the climax of the illness. For this reason the physician should know beforehand when the crisis will happen, and the patient can [then] be asked to rest and repose [until the predicted critical day]. On that day one should not give him any medicine nor let him exercise strenuously, but one should let nature alone and in peace so that it can complete its activity and its combat against the illness. One should not disturb [nature] with anything that might affect it or by anything that the patient takes upon himself. Hippocrates has said that if you think it good [that the patient] exercises a little bit while the illness is still in the beginning, let him exercise, but if the illness has reached its climax it is better to leave the patient resting and at ease.

[10] The regimen of food during a crisis and the knowledge of the days of a crisis: The physician should [know about] these for the treatment of the patient and his nutrition. When the [illness] approaches its climax food should not be a heavy burden for nature, because in that case nature would have to divide its activity and occupy itself both with breaking up the food that [the patient] takes and with [fighting] the causes of the illness. Therefore [the patient] should have an extremely thinning regimen when the illness is at its climax. It makes no difference whether you say "at the climax of the illness" or you say "with regard to the causes of the complete, finished illness".

[11] The climax of an illness varies. It can occur already on the fourth day; in that case, the patient should have an extremely thinning regimen from the beginning [of the illness], that is, he should totally abstain from food.[14] When[15] the climax of the illness is delayed until the seventh day, the patient needs a regimen that is thinning, but not extremely so; and he should feed himself initially with barley gruel or honey water. If the climax of the illness is delayed until the fourteenth day the patient should be fed with egg yolk or

14 Cf. Hippocrates, *Aphorisms* 1.7-11 (pp. 102-105); and CG 294-298 (K 884.8-14; 885.17-886.2). Here again the author of this summary has placed materials from book II near the beginning; as noted in the introduction, this version of the summary exhibits the most radical reorganization of material.

15 Cf. CG 296-297 (K 884.15-18).

with some crumbs of clean [i.e. made from refined flour] bread. Hippocrates[16] has said that when the fever is high, pains will appear that are extremely severe; then an extremely thinning regimen must be employed. If this is not the case, it is possible to employ a more thickening regimen. When the illness is more severe and more remote from its climax, one should increase [the amount of] food a little bit, and when it reaches its climax or a short time before that one should diminish [the amount of] food.

[12] The good crisis and the bad crisis:[17] If the limit of the climax of a certain type of illness and its motion—whether it belongs to the illnesses that are considered to be acute in a general sense—is known, and so also if the illness moves in an inappropriately fast or slow motion; then, if you look at the [rate of] increase of the illness and of the concoction at a time of warning as well as the symptoms that occur before the crisis, you will have an indication for the fast or slow [motion] of the illness. If these symptoms were preceded by good symptoms that indicate safety and concoction, you should know that the crisis will be good and safe. But if these symptoms are preceded by bad symptoms, and they have not been preceded by signs of coction, you should know that the crisis will be bad.

[13] Afterwards (after paying attention to all of the signs described in the preceding passage) you will realize that knowledge in the matter of the crisis is something that is necessary for the prognosis, with regard to estimating the nutrition [of the patient] and for every single thing you have to do at any time in accordance with that knowledge. Just as signs can be seen in the world from which one can derive what will happen and which indicate the occurrence of that event and limit the time of its occurrence, be they signs that are seen in this world or [those that are seen] in the positions of the stars—so also signs from nature are visible in the urine and arterial pulse and stool which indicate whether the outcome of the activity of nature in its fight with the illness will be good or bad. The days in which those signs can be seen are called the days of warning[18] and of observation.[19]

---

16 Cf Hippocrates, *Aphorisms* 1.7 (pp. 102-103): "When the disease is very acute, immediately, not only is the pain extreme, but also it is essential to employ a regimen of extreme strictness".

17 These subheadings are another sign of the reorganization characteristic of this version of the summaries.

18 "Days of indication and observation"; Hebrew ימי הבשורה והמבט reflects the Greek "ἐπιδήλοις τε καὶ θεωρηταῖς ἡμέραις (Galen, *De crisibus* (K 9.809.13-14; Ḥunayn (CG 169, l. 5): في الأيام المنذرة ("the indicator days," trans. Cooper). Note that Ḥunayn does not translate Greek θεωρηταῖς (CG 168, n. 283: "and to be watched).

19 This passage sums up succinctly the arguments for the utility of knowing the critical

[14] The days of warning and the days of observation: Just as not all days are days of crisis, so [also] not all days are days of warning. However,[20] if the seventh day is the day of the crisis then the fourth day is the day of the warning, for if one sees a cloud floating on top of the urine or suspended in it on the fourth day, the crisis will without any doubt be on the seventh day. Every[21] week can be divided into two [equal] parts whereby the division falls on the fourth day. The fourth day of every week shows what will happen on the seventh day, because it (i.e. the fourth day) divides the week into two parts. Likewise, if the crisis comes on the fourteenth day, the eleventh day warns of it. Hippocrates[22] intended this matter when he said that the calculation of the critical days is by increments of four each until the twentieth [day]. When the days of warning transform into critical days, then the indications that indicate them fall on other preceding days.[23] When the days of warning have passed beyond the twentieth day, the periods of their warning become longer, as they warn in weeks until the fortieth day.

[15] The critical days are known from what has been noticed and observed repeatedly, namely that the functioning[24] of nearly everything that belongs to the world of coming into being and passing away follows the course of the moon. One's judgment should therefore be in accordance with this [principle]. It has already been observed and noticed regarding the days of crisis that the seventh and fourteenth [day] are the most excellent critical days, while the sixth day is the worst of the critical days. A crisis on this day always comes with hardness and strong agitation and sometimes it leads to an increase [in the disease] or an inflammation affecting one of the organs. A crisis in which the patient is affected by another [kind of] struggle is also not good: and when there is sweating on the sixth day it is not equal and not over the whole body.[25]

---

days; note the analogies to other fields of medicine (uroscopy) and sciences (astral prognostication).

20 Cf. CG. 124-5 (K 784.11-16).

21 Cf. CG. 234-5 (K 845.14-17).

22 Cf. Hippocrates, *Prognostics II* (Loeb Classical Library, London 1923, repr. 1981), 20 (pp. 42-43): "So in the most acute diseases keep on adding periods of four days, up to twenty, to find the time when the attacks end"; CG 274-275.

23 I.e., the crisis will move back to day four or day eleven.

24 We translate according to its context the Hebrew term שמוש, literally "service". Here it refers to the way things behave in their natural course, especially when this is cyclical; things that rise and fall, increase and decrease. They grossly follow the moon, i.e. increasing for about two weeks, then decreasing for about two weeks.

25 Does this mean that the patient on day six is "busy" with something else and not free

[16] The shift of a crisis, its exceeding its limit, and coming after its limit: When a crisis exceeds [its limit] and comes earlier or later, it has many causes. The first and most powerful [of these are] causes [affecting] that which falls under the category of coming to be and passing away, even if they are the heavenly motions. Their circuit is known and they must be orderly, and so they set the flow of nature in cycles, but none of them is free of deviation[26]. True, the most part of it (nature) must be orderly [even] with regard to that which falls under [the category] of coming to be and passing away, but it is [still] only mostly so, not such as to mandate its always being in the same way.[27] It is possible that nature awakens to repel that which is harmful to it before the right time to do so either because it is extensive or because it is severe. In general, the effective cause is because of haste, just like a soldier who is triggered by some of his limbs to do battle before the proper time. But it is also possible that the patient commits a mistake against himself and this mistake is the cause of the deviation of the crisis from its [proper] time. It is also possible that this happens because of a mistake by someone else, for instance by the physician who is charged with his cure or [that it is caused] by external causes, such as phlegm or exertion, or worry, or insomnia, or fear, or because of a change in the weather. Accordingly, Hippocrates[28] said that a doctor should not restrict himself to do what is required without the help of the patient himself, of the attendants and of external [factors].

[17] Sometimes[29] we attribute the crisis to the wrong day because we did not know when the illness began, and we [mistakenly] took it to be when the patient takes to his bed. However,[30] the [real] time of its beginning is that of the beginning of the fever. Many people are affected by an illness and are forced by circumstances to do what they were used to do when they were healthy. Sometimes nature is not capable of expelling the dis-

to deal with the crisis?

26 A difficult and cumbersome sentence. The intent seems to be that even the most orderly of causes, i.e. the regular circuits of the heavenly bodies, is not free of some anomaly.

27 The discussion of the causes of error or mistake in the critical days, something that occupies Galen's attention quite a bit in *On Critical Days*, is here preceded by a general remark on regularity and order in nature.

28 Cf. Hippocrates, *Aphorisms* 1.1 (pp. 98-99); CG 196-7 (K 825.3-5).

29 "Sometimes…bed": cf. CG 144-145 (K 796.9-16).

30 Cf. Ḥunayn, trans. Cooper, CG 146-7 (K 797.11-13): "For we must count the beginning of an illness to be this time when the fever begins in an obvious manner, to the point that the patient is forced to take to his bed".

ease in its totality on one day, so that it is forced to postpone it to another day. Then the crisis is attributed to the second day, as in the case of the crisis that is on the seventh day, but nature is not strong enough to repel the disease completely on that day; instead it is forced to repel the remnant [of the illness] on the eighth day and, consequently, the crisis is attributed to the eighth [day]. Sometimes fevers have cycles that come in pairs, as happens in the case of the double[31] quartan [fever]. An illness may also have its normal crisis on the seventh or ninth day, with a high fever occurring on the eighth or sixth day, for which reason nature is restrained from beginning to expel that which is already prepared to be expelled, even though its preparation [for expulsion] has been completed. For all these reasons a crisis may fall on other days [than it normally falls on] and the limit of the real critical day is corrupted.

[18][32] The complete crisis and the defective crisis: A crisis should have the following characteristics: it should be complete, trustworthy and reliable on the day of the crisis, distinct, and have a day that warns of it. A bad, defective crisis has the opposite of these [characteristics]. A complete crisis is a crisis in which the illness is completely resolved so that no trace of its causes is left in the body. A trustworthy[33] crisis is a crisis that one can trust that it will not return. This [crisis] is also called true and reliable and not dangerous. A crisis is trustworthy when it is preceded by signs of concoction and when they occur on a reliable critical day. A safe[34] crisis is a crisis in which there are no dangerous symptoms in it as, for instance palpitations, intestinal pains and the like. A distinct crisis is a crisis in which the factors that determine the end of the illness are distinct [and] clear, such as sweat, diarrhea and the like. A crisis for which warning has been given is a crisis that is preceded by its signs on one of its warning days. For nature does not approach illnesses all of a sudden but deals with them slowly until it overcomes them. So when it moves on them, it repels them by means of the warning days.[35] Now I will mention the different critical days.

---

31 In which paroxysms of fever occur in a repeating pattern of 2 consecutive days followed by 1 day of remission.

32 Cf. CG 108-111, ll. (K 776.6-17).

33 "trustworthy" (שמור); cf. Ḥunayn, CG 108-9, l. 15 (K 776.13): صحيح; (trustworthy, trans. Cooper).

34 "safe" (בטוח); cf. Ḥunayn, CG 108-9, l. 16 (K 776.14-15): سليم.

35 Very unclear; seems to mean that though nature rises up against illness only slowly, the warning days show that nature is actively involved in the process of healing.

[19] Book two: The[36] critical days and their classification: Some critical days are strongest and best, and they are the seventh and fourteenth day, for these are the best and most trustworthy critical days between the beginning of the illness and the twentieth day. The secondary days that come after them: These are the days that warn of them, i.e. the fourth, the eleventh and the seventeenth day. The tertiary days that come after them: those are the days in which the crisis comes earlier or later; of the fourth day it is the third and fifth day, and of the seventh day it is the sixth and eighth day. When the crisis that occurs on the eleventh day comes earlier it will for the most part come on the ninth day because of the urging of the power of the fever. These are the days on which a good crisis happens in most cases. The sixth day also belongs to these days. However, the seventh day attracts as it were its power and rules over it. And[37] the crisis that occurs [on the sixth day] is not safe and not complete, because the sweat will not pour forth [over the body] equally. It will not turn out like the crisis that has the strength of [a crisis on day] seven, which governs like a good king; the status of the [crisis on] day six is that of an evil tyrant.[38] A crisis occurring on the twentieth day cannot come on the twenty-first, unless it has been warned of (?). If this is the case then the warning day is the eighteenth. However, the thirteenth day is totally unlike the days on which the crisis occurs, because it is the most impotent of all critical days. The second day does not have a crisis in any way because its (i.e. nature's) strength is still strong enough to endure the harm done to it, so it is not stimulated before the proper time.

[20] The [critical] days on which a crisis does not occur and does not happen in any respect are the fifteenth, sixteenth and nineteenth day. For the fifteenth day comes after the fourteenth, the sixteenth day precedes the seventeenth, and the nineteenth day precedes the twentieth day. Weeks in which a critical day occurs are counted as overlapping[39] or as separate.

[21] The separation between the weeks and the cycle of the four warning [days]: The best [weeks counted] as separate are the first and the second week, while the best weeks [counted] as overlapping are the second and third, for according to the calculation of the days of the week from the fourteenth day the critical day is not the twenty-first, but rather the twentieth

36 "The critical days...the sixth and eighth day"; cf. CG 238-9 (K 847.6-17).

37 Cf. Ḥunayn, trans. Cooper (CG 126-7, ll. 10-11 (K 786.1-2)): "If he breaks into a sweat, then it will not quite cover his whole body uniformly with heat".

38 Cf. CG 128-9, ll. 7-8 (K 786.17.1-2).

39 "overlapping"; cf. Cooper, CG 75: "here means that the end day of the first period is the same as the first day of the next period"; see as well ibid., 244-245, ll. 3-5 (K 850.16-851.2).

day, as the fourteenth day is the beginning of the third week. Likewise the calculation of the days that are counted according to the cycle of the four indicators of the crisis occurring in weeks is like the calculation of the weeks. The most severe critical day in terms of agitation and hardness will be one [that occurs up to day] fourteen; the crisis at this time comes with hardness and agitation. So also the critical days that fall between those days [that have been mentioned] will happen in accordance with the computation of cycles. None (i.e. no warning) will fall after the fourteenth, not to mention (?) the twentieth. Thus the warning days that are on the computation of the fourteenth are weak, because the indication for this day is [only] by weeks.[40] So also the cycles of weeks after the fortieth day are weak, because the movement will then be every twenty [days]. Thus [the indication will be] that the crisis is on days forty, sixty, eighty, one hundred, and one hundred and twenty. The crisis can come even later, in keeping with the same [arithmetic] series.

[22] Hippocrates[41] has said that the summer illnesses resolve in winter and the winter illnesses – in the summer. He has related that there are crises that have cycles that are more remote[42] than these. He[43] said that in the case of many children's diseases, some terminate after seventy [days], some after seven months, some after seven years, and some when they reach puberty. And in the book *Epidemics*,[44] as this book was his casebook, he mentions all the days on which a crisis occurs, that is to say the days whose nature is characterized by the crisis and the days which tend by the force of the crisis to the day on which it occurs first.

[23] In the *Aphorisms* and *Prognostics* he mentions the days on which a crisis occurs because it is specific to their nature. In[45] the first book of *Epi-*

---

40 That is to say, warning by weeks is less precise and useful than a warning of two or three days, as in a good crisis.

41 Cf. *Epidemics* (Loeb Classical Library, London 1994), 3.15 (pp. 254-5); cf. CG 294-5, ll. 8-10 (K 883.16- 884.1).

42 I.e., they resolve only after a longer period of time.

43 Cf. *Aphorisms* 3.28, p. 133: "Most diseases of children reach a crisis in forty days, in seven months, in seven years, at the approach of puberty.

44 I.e., *Epidemics*, book 1; cf. Ḥunayn, trans. Cooper, CG 118-9, ll.1-4 (K 780.18-781.4): "What points me to this is the fact that he must have been guided by it in the first book of his *Epidemics* treatise, in which he enumerated many of the critical days, and he returned to mention some of them in the *Prognostics*, and in the *Aphorisms*" (trans. Cooper) and CG 276-7, ll. 2-3 (K 871.9-10): "In the first book of the *Epidemics*, he counted all of the critical days in order" (trans. Cooper).

45 Cf. CG 276-7, ll. 1-9 (K 871.9-14).

demics he mentions regarding the critical days the even [days], namely the fourth, sixth, eighth, fourteenth, eighteenth, thirty-fourth, fortieth, sixtieth, eightieth, one hundredth and one hundred and twentieth [day]. Of the odd [days] he mentions the third, fifth, seventh, ninth, eleventh, seventeenth, twenty-first and thirty-first. In[46] the *Aphorisms* and *Prognostics* he states that the crisis necessarily occurs in [series of] sevens and fours. In[47] the *Aphorisms*[48] he remarks that in acute diseases the crisis comes within fourteen days, and that the fourth day warns of the seventh; and that the second week begins from the eighth day and that the eleventh day is warned by it, because this day is the[49] warning day of the second week. Moreover, the seventeenth day is the warning day of the third week because it is the fourth day from the fourteenth day and the seventh from the eleventh [day].

[24] However, in the *Prognostics*[50] he said that the fevers culminate on[51] the same days, both those from which patients recover and those from which they die. For the fever that is safest and has the most trustworthy signs will abate on the fourth day or before it, and the most malignant fever with the worst symptoms will kill on the fourth day or before it. The first period [of fevers] ends here. The second period ends in the seventh day, and the third period ends in the eleventh day, and the fourth period ends in the fourteenth day, and the fifth period ends in the seventeenth day, and the sixth period ends in the twentieth day. The[52] increments of these periods continue up to the twentieth day. It is impossible for any of these [periods] to be counted by whole days, as it is impossible for the year and the months to be counted by whole days.[53] Thereafter,[54] according to this pattern [and]

---

46 Cf. CG 270-1, ll. 9-11 (K 868.11-15).

47 Cf. CG 274-5, ll. 9-16 (K 871.1-5).

48 Cf. *Aphorisms* 2.24 (pp. 114-5).

49 "the warning day"; cf. *Aphorisms* 2.24 (pp. 114-5): ἡ τέταρτη (the fourth day; trans. Jones); Ḥunayn, CG 274-5 (l. 14): الرابع (K 871.4).

50 Cf. *Prognostics* 20, ll. 1-22 (pp. 42-43); CG 274-5, ll. 3-11 (K 870.1-16).

51 "on the same days": lit. "in the numbers of the same days".

52 "The increments of these periods continue up to the twentieth day"; cf. *Prognostics* 20, ll. cf. Ḥunayn; CG 274, ll. 7-8): وهذه الزيادات تكون في أربعة أربعة في الأمراض الحادّة إلى العشرين (And these increments are by four-day intervals in acute illnesses up to the twentieth day) (= *Prognostics* 20, ll. 13-15).

53 "days": Ḥunayn adds: لا كسر فيها cf. CG 274-5, ll. 8-9 (without fractions; trans. Cooper).

54 Cf. Ḥunayn, CG 274-5, ll. 9-10: ثمّ من بعد ذلك على النظام وهذه الزيادات الدور الأوّل اليوم الرابع والثلثين ("And (the counting proceeds) thereafter according to this pattern, and these increments. The first period is the thirty-fourth day" (trans. Cooper); cf. note 805 (Cooper): "I am still unsure why the thirty-fourth day is important here. The scribe of L had problems with this also, and his text adds the twenty-fourth and twenty-eighth days to

these increments, is the first period the thirty-fourth day. And the second period [ends][55] on the fortieth day, and the third on the sixtieth day.

[25] He said that the cause of the third week [ending on the twentieth day] is in accordance with the causes of overlapping, since the computation of the month is not in whole and complete days.[56] For the greatest natural principle is this: what is in heaven effects what happens on earth, especially the moon, because of all the heavenly bodies, it is closest to the earth. The motion of the moon is not its revolution that is joined to the sun (i.e. the synodic month), which is approximately twenty-nine [days], but rather its revolution in the ecliptic (i.e. the sidereal month) which is 27 ⅓ days. And since these days are divided into four quarters [and] because the quarters of the moon, when taken relative to the ecliptic are stronger (i.e. larger)-- and they are not divided relative to the revolution of the moon until it joins with the sun (the synodic month, which is longer, so each quarter would be longer and hence weaker)—so the quarter is 6 + ½ + ⅓ days.[57] Accordingly the third week ends on the twentieth day and not on the twenty-first day. The second week ends on the fourteenth day. He counts the twentieth day as a critical day because its half begins on the last day of the third week, and the crisis fights for half [of the day]. It is now time to relate the causes of the critical days.

[26] Book Three. He said that Pythagoras and his circle ascribe the causes of the critical days to the numbers. They held it to be necessary that whatever stars revolve in the heavens possess effects, in accordance with the attendant changes in their configurations. Together with this, they held it to be necessary that the number that follows upon the cycles of what comes to be, as we have explained, has a power by means of which seasonal periods

---

this first period. One possibility is that the thirty-fourth day is twenty plus fourteen, or the major fourteenth day period within the second twenty-day cycle".

55 "[ends]": cf. Cf. Ḥunayn, CG 274-5, l. 10: ينتهي.

56 Cf. *Prognostics* 20, ll. 15-18: "None of them, however, can be exactly calculated in whole days; neither can whole days be used to measure the solar year and the lunar month" (trans. Jones); CG 366-7; ll. 2-4.

57 The word order in this sentence has been rearranged for purposes of clarity. The information conveyed here is simply this: For purposes of reckoning critical days, the moon's sidereal period, rather than its synodic period, is employed. The sidereal period is shorter, so each quarter is shorter, hence stronger, in the sense that a shorter period of time is needed for a cycle (measured as a quarter revolution). 6 + ½ + ⅓ is the standard way of writing out fractions in the period; in our decimal notation, we would write 6.83.

come about in that which comes about.[58] That is to say, they thought it not be in vain that the worlds are three, i.e., the unchanging world, the limited world, and the world that lies beneath the moon.[59] Rather, the reason for this is that the number three is primary, and so the worlds were divided up in this way. For this very reason each of the species has one of the numbers especially [associated] with it. Were it not so, what is the rationale for acute diseases terminating in multiples of four and seven, and chronic diseases terminating every twenty days, unless it be the case that what is necessary for the orb (it must move in regular cycles, on account of the numbers associated with it?) is also necessary for that which moves in an unnatural fashion? All the more so, [since this usually happens?] without anomalous measures (i.e., though disease is unnatural, its cycles still follow regular patterns, in general)? For this reason,[60] days six and eight, which fall together (are classified together?) with regard to fever, have the worst crises.

[27] But for Galen, number is a representation [or: likeness] that a person thinks in his mind. He does not consider it to have being, or reality, and to exist as a principle.[61] For this reason, he scorned many treatises of Aristo-

58 This last sentence appears in a horrific Hebrew with numerous variants; we have tried to make as best sense of it as possible. The key point, if our understanding is correct, is that for these Pythagoreans, the heavens rather than numbers are the primary causes for terrestrial processes. (As we shall see in the following sentence, number is the cause for the division of reality into three "worlds", with the heavens being above the earth.) In line with the principle stated in [25], they too subscribe to the rule that the greatest cause of all for terrestrial events is the heavens. However, terrestrial events—whose primary cause is the changing stellar configuration—happen in measured cycles, and the numbers associated with these cycles have a power of their own.

59 The idea calls to mind the discussion in Aristotle's *Physics*, III.4, 203a 4-17. Aristotle takes up together the theories of Plato and the Pythagoreans, pointing to the differences between them. On the admittedly flimsy basis of this one sentence in our text, it seems that the Summaries are confronting an original amalgam of the two: a fixed, presumably unlimited world beyond the heavens; the limited celestial world; and the sublunar realm. On the notions of limited and unlimited, see Walter Burkert, *Lore and Science in Ancient Pythagoreanism*, (Cambridge MA 1972), p. 258. In particular, we have here a fairly standard neoplatonic classification of three worlds: the highest, unchanging world; then the celestial realm; and the sublunar realm. Support for this interpretation can be drawn from a miscopy in Paris 884, a manuscript whose readings we have generally not included in the apparatus. For the first world, in place of הקיים, Paris 884 displays השפלים, "the baser things", which makes no sense. This is easily seen to be a miscopy for השכלים, "the intellects", yielding the widespread classification into worlds of the intellects, heavenly bodies, and terrestrial bodies.

60 Following the reading in Paris 884.

61 The Hebrew philosophical terminology has been translated according to the context.

tle's followers, who are linked to the Peripatetics, saying that it is the same whether we say that the seventh day is the critical day or that the gates of the city of Thebes are seven.[62]

[28] So the seventh day was a critical day in the place of the number seven.[63] The issue of crisis connects only to the configurations of the moon. He thinks that the risings and configurations of all the stars produce effects upon us; but (?) their actions are not in general things, such as those that come about in summer and winter. Instead, their actions are in particular things. However, the moon's actions are of two kinds. One of them is in its motion until it joins [again] with the sun, the other in its motion in its circuit in the ecliptic. The circuit of the moon until it catches up with the sun is in twenty-nine and one half days; but the time in which the moon makes one revolution in the ecliptic is twenty-seven and one-third days. They say that the configurations of the moon vis-à-vis the sun produce general effects. The configurations vis-à-vis its circle (circuit?) in the ecliptic produce effects of a more particular sort than the former. The strongest configuration of the moon are those of the half circuit, and they are those in which the sun is at its maximum elongation. After them come the configurations in which

---

Ha'amadah has been rendered "being" and *qiyyum* "reality". Semantically, both convey the sense of "standing", and thus are appropriate for the notion of a self-standing entity or substance (and not far removed at all semantically form the concept of *hypostasis*). The Hebrew *dimuy*, "representation" or "likeness" (cf. Mauro Zonta, *Un dizionario filosofico ebraico del XIII secolo. L'introduzione al* "Sefer De'ot ha-Filosofim" di Shem Tob ibn Falaquera (Torino 1992), 62-64), cannot be the Arabic *muthul* (plural of *mithāl*, but in this context always appearing in the plural), in the sense of Platonic idea, since Galen rejects the reality of these. Moreover, in the second of his lists of Pythagorean terminology, which is displayed as part of Galen's stern rejection of Pythagorean arithmology, the monad is identified with ἰδέα. Clearly the authors are struggling to express as clearly as possible the difference between the Pythagoreans, who hold number to be a self-standing, actual entity, like a Platonic idea, and Galen, who does not. The passage before us echoes discussions in Aristotle and especially later Academicians, such as Speusippus, which treat together the Platonic ideas (Arabic *muthul*) and Pythagorean number theory; the key texts are Aristotle's *Metaphysics*, beginnings of Books XII and XIII.

62 This passage is very obscure in the Hebrew, displaying very well the wear and tear of crossing linguistic, cultural, and historical boundaries from Greek (referring here to the Greek philosophical vocabulary that was used to express this brand of philosophy, even if there was no Greek *Vorlage* for the Summaries), to Syriac (most likely), to Arabic, to Hebrew; see the discussion in Langermann, "Astral Connections", 107.

63 Another unclear sentence. It seems to say that the seventh day, i.e., the lapse of seven days, rather than the number seven, is the cause of the crisis on that day.

the moon has two boundaries (i.e., half moon, with moon bounded by a semi-circle and a straight line, and gibbous moon, bounded by two arcs). The weakest configuration is that which the moon has at its first rising. Moreover, the beginning of the revolution of the moon in its circuit in the ecliptic is [analogous to] the day on which the illness began. In keeping with this analogy one ought to observe and compute the cycles.

[29] However, we do not accept Galen's statement that during the three days during which the moon is not seen, the moon produces no effect on earth; and for that reason, it joins to the closest thing, [which is] the motion of the moon until it catches up with the sun in its orb in the ecliptic orb. For this does not necessarily follow from [the observation] that no winds blow when the moon is hidden, and that they blow when it is revealed.[64]

[30] The effect of the moon on earth. It is, however, fitting that we accept from him what he said, and he said it well, that the effects of the moon in the computation of the illness should be relative to its circuit in the ecliptic; but it varies in keeping with its configurations relative to the sun. That is to say, the quarter[65] of the moon acts not just relative to the illness but also relative to the sun. So also with regard to the configurations relative to the other stars and their motion: when it arrives at the termination in one of the illnesses, one finds there a shift from one thing to another. Likewise with regard to the risings and settings of the well-known stars. In line with this Hippocrates said that drinking a medicine before the rising of Sirius as well as after its rising is difficult.[66]

---

64 Yet another unclear sentence. During the days of the moon's invisibility, it is catching up with the sun and passing it. In K 907.5-7 (cf. CG 332), Galen says that for a period of three days, the moon may or may not be seen (that is, it will surely not be seen for at least or day or two, but it may be briefly seen on the third day), but either way, it is not powerful enough to effect any change on earth. There is a brief reference to the stopping (*stasis*) of winds at the end of K 908 (CG 334) but it is not clear what Galen wishes to conclude from this. In any event, the authors of these Summaries read Galen as concluding that the moon has no effect during the three days of its invisibility. Perhaps this justifies speaking of four units of seven days, since 28 days is close to the length of the sidereal month, and allows one to finesse the longer synodic month which includes a short stint of lunar impotence. This seems to be the intent of the beginning of the passage that follows. But this passage remains obscure.

65 Hebrew רבוע, literally "squaring" or "quadrature", but here seems to be a miscopy. The quarters of the lunar cycle (both synodic and sidereal) are approximately seven days, just like the "default" cycle of the crisis.

66 We have not been able to locate this exact statement in the Hippocratic corpus. However, Hippocrates does warn us to guard against the risings of the stars, for example in *Epidemics* I.11; for a fuller discussion of this passage, see Langermann, "Astral Connec-

[31] The risings and settings of the stars should not by themselves be taken as signs for the seasons of the year and what comes to be in them, because they also produce effects in inanimate beings. Among these [considerations? astral connection of disease?] is the sun's reversal at the summer solstice, and the days following the rising of Arcturus, when there are no red bile fevers because its rising has a power that sifts them out, as Theophrastus said.[67] But the changes that follow the months come to be along with the [cycle of] the moon, as is shown by sea creatures, especially the sea-urchin.[68] That is to say that this animal moves along with the moon, growing larger and smaller together with it. Epilepsy also has fits in keeping with the count of the moon (lit. month) at the time of its waning. The distance of the moon, such as it is in keeping with a count analogous to the month, [is the cause?] for the blowing of winds that begin to blow with the rising of the moon and shift, then changing at half moon. And the winds that come to be at half moon, change when it becomes full. And the winds that blow when it is full, change when it is once again half moon. And so Aristotle said.[69]

[32] Thus it has been shown that it is proper to ascribe great power to day seven and day fourteen, since quadrature and opposition are at those configurations. Now the configuration that the moon has on its rising ends on the fourth [day]; so also the configuration with a double boundary, which is at trine and is in service until the eleventh [day]. Because the sun has its effect on generation, its changes will be over boundaries (bounded periods of time) that are larger. The summaries of the third book of the treatise *On Critical Days* by Galen are done, and with their completion the treatise is complete, thank God.

---

tion", 109-110.

67 Another difficult paragraph; cf. Langermann, "Astral Connection", 109-11. 'Theophrastus' is a good surmise for the name intended by the Hebrew letter chain B'WQRSṬ'S. Theophrastus has something to say about risings and settings in his *On Weather Signs* (Arthur Hort, *Theophrastus, Inquiry into Plants and Minor Works* (London 1916), 2: 390-97), but not the connection between Arcturus and red bile fever.

68 Literally, "the animal that is covered by shards".

69 Aristotle speaks of the connection between winds and the moon's phases in *Generation of Animals II*, 4.738a 22-3; see Langermann, "Astral Connection", 109.

Bibliography

Anawati, Georges C. *Rasā'il ibn Rushd al-Ṭibbīyah*. Cairo, repr. 2005.

Averroes: Obra Medica, trad. Maria Concepción Vázquez de Benito. Seville and Malaga 1998, limited edition.

Bergsträsser, G. *Ḥunain ibn Isḥâq über die syrischen und arabischen Galen-Übersetzungen* (Abhandlungen für die Kunde des Morgenlandes, XVII, 2; Leipzig 1925).

Bos, Gerrit. "Maimonides on Medicinal Measures and Weights." Aleph 9 (2009): 255-276.

———, *Novel Medical and General Hebrew Terminology from the 13th Century*. Vol. 2. *Journal of Semitic Studies*, Suppl. 30 (Oxford, 2013)

Bos, Gerrit and Y. Tzvi Langermann. "An Unknown Summary of Galen's *On the Elements According to Hippocrates*, attributed to Ḥunayn Ibn Isḥāq." Forthcoming in *Arabic Sciences and Philosophy*.

Boyle, C. (ed.). *Medieval Prognosis and Astrology: A Working Edition of the Aggregationes de crisi et creticis diebus: with Introduction and English Summary*. Cambridge 1991.

Brockelmann, C. *Lexicon Syriacum*. Halle 1928.

Burkert, Walter. *Lore and Science in Ancient Pythagoreanism*. Cambridge MA 1972.

Bylebyl, Jerome J. and Walter Pagel. "The chequered career of Galen's doctrine on the pulmonary veins." *Medical History* 15 (1971): 211-229.

Cooper, C.M. *Galen*, De diebus decretoriis, *from Greek into Arabic. A Critical Edition, with Translation and Commentary, of Ḥunayn Ibn Isḥāq*, Kitāb ayyām al-buḥrān. Farnham-Burlington 2011.

Dietrich, Albrecht. *Medicinalia Arabica: Studien uber arabische medizinische Handschriften in turkischen und syrischen Bibliotheken*. Göttingen 1966.

Galen. *Über die Arten der Fieber in der arabischen Version des Ḥunain ibn Isḥāq*. Ed. and trans. Matthias Werhard. Inaugural-Dissertation Ludwig-Maximilians-Universität, Munich 2004.

Garofalo, I. "La traduzione araba de de temperamentis, del de optima constitutione e del de bono habitu." In: V. Boudon-Millot et al. (eds.). *Ecdotica e ricezione dei testi medici*. Naples 2006, 125–135.

———, "La traduzione araba del commento di Ioannes Grammatikos al De pulsibus di Galeno." In: A. Garyza and J. Jouanna (eds.). *I testi medici greci, tradizione e ecdotica. Atti del III Convegno Internazionale, Napoli 15–18 ottobre 1997*. Naples 1999, 185–218.

Gutas, Dimitri. *Greek Thought, Arabic Culture: The Graeco-Arabic Translation Movement in Baghdad and Early 'Abbasid Society (2nd-4th/5th-10th c.)*. London 2012.

———, "Paul the Persian on the classification of the parts of Aristotle's philosophy: a milestone between Alexandria and Baġdâd." *Der Islam 60* (1983): 231-267.

Hippocrates. *Aphorisms*. Loeb Classical Library, London 1931, repr. 1979.

———, *Prognostics II*. Loeb Classical Library, London 1923, repr. 1981.

———, *Epidemics*. Loeb Classical Library, London 1994.

———, *Crises*. Loeb Classical Library, London 2010.

Hort, Arthur. *Theophrastus, Inquiry into Plants and Minor Works*. London 1916.

Ibn Juljul. *Ṭabaqāt al-aṭibbā' wa-'l-ḥukamā'*. Second printing, Beirut 1985.

Irvine, J.T. and O. Temkin. "Who was Akilaos?" *Bulletin of the History of Medicine 77* (2003): 12-24.

Iskandar, A.Z. "An attempted reconstruction of the late Alexandrian medical curriculum." *Medical History 20* (1976): 235-258.

———,"Bibliographical studies in medical and scientific Arabic works. Galen's *fī 'Amal al-tashrīḥ* (On Anatomical procedures), the Alexandrian book entitled *fī 'l-Tashrīḥ ilā ‹l-muta'allimīn* (On Anatomy for students), and Rhazes' *al-Kāfī fī 'l-ṭibb* (The Sufficient Book on Medicine)." *Oriens 25-26* (1976): 133-147.

Klatzkin, Jacob. *Thesaurus Philosophicus Linguae Hebraicae*. New York 1968.

Kühn, C.G. *Claudii Galeni Opera Omnia*, 20 vols. Leipzig 1821-1833, repr. Hildesheim 1967.

Lameer, Joep. "From Alexandria to Baghdad: Reflections on the Genesis of a Problematical Tradition." In Remke Kruk and Gerhard Endress (eds.). *The Ancient Tradition in Christian and Islamic Hellenism. Studies on the transmission of Greek philosophy and sciences dedicated to H.J. Drossaart Lulofs on his ninetieth birthday* (= CNWS Publications 50). Leiden 1997, 181-191.

Langermann, Y. Tzvi. "Maimonides on the Synochous Fever." *Israel Oriental Studies 12* (1993): 175-198.

———, "The Astral Connections of Critical Days: Some Late Antique Sources Preserved in Hebrew and Arabic." In Anna Akasoy, Charles Burnett and Ronit Yoeli-Tlalim (eds.). *Astromedicine, Astrology, and Medicine, East and West*. Florence 2008, 99-118.

———, "Islamic Atomism and the Galenic Tradition." *History of Science 47* (2009): 277-295.

———, "Critical Notes on a Study of Galen's On Critical Days, or A Study in Need of Critical Repairs." *Aestimatio 9* (2012): 220-240.

Liddell, H.G. and R. Scott. *A Greek English Lexicon*. Repr. Oxford 1989.

Lieber, E. "Galen in Hebrew: the transmission of Galen's works in the medieval Islamic world." In: V. Nutton (ed.). *Galen: Problems and Prospects*. London, 1981, 167-186.

Maimonides. *Medical Aphorisms, Treatises 1-5*, ed. and trans. Gerrit Bos. Provo 2004.

Meyerhof, Max. "New light on Ḥunain Ibn Isḥâq and his period." *Isis 8* (1926): 685-724.

———, *Von Alexandrien nach Bagdad: Ein Beitrag zur Geschichte des philosophischen und medizinischen Unterrichts bei den Arabern*. Berlin 1930.

Pormann, P.E. "The Alexandrian Summary (*Jawāmiʿ*) of Galen's *On the Sects for Beginners*: Commentary or Abridgement?" *Bulletin of the Institute of Classical Studies* 47 (2004): 11-33.

———, "Jean le grammarien et le De sectis dans la littérature médicale d'Alexandrie." In Ivan Garofalo and Amneris Roselli (eds.). *Galenismo e medicina tardoantica: fonti greche, latine e arabe*. Naples 2003, 197-248.

Richler, B. *Hebrew Manuscripts in the Biblioteca Palatina in Parma. Catalogue. Palaegraphical and codicological descriptions:* Malachi Beit-Arié. Jerusalem 2001.

Sālim, Muḥammad Salīm. *Kitāb Jālīnūs fī Firaq al-ṭibb lil-mutaʿallimīn* (Muntakhabāt al-Iskandarāniyyīn 1). Cairo 1977.

———, *Kitāb Jālīnūs ilā Ghulūqūn fī al-Taʿattī li-shifāʾ al-amrāḍ*. Cairo 1982.

———, *Kitāb Jālīnūs ilā Ṭutrūn fī al-nabḍ lil-mutaʿalimīn*. Cairo 1985.

———, *Kitāb Jālīnūs fī al-usṭuqusāt ʿalā raʾy Abuqrāṭ naql Abī Zayd Ḥunayn b. Isḥāq al-ʿIbādī al-mutaṭabbib* (Muntakhabāt al-Iskandarāniyyīn 5). Cairo 1986.

Savage-Smith, E. "Galen's lost ophthalmology and the 'Summaria Alexandrinorum'." In: V. Nutton (ed.). *The unknown Galen*. London, 2002, 121-138.

Schacht, Joseph and Max Meyerhof. "Maimonides Against Galen: On Philosophy and Cosmogony." *Bulletin of the Faculty of Arts of the University of Egypt* 5 (1937): 53-88 (Arabic section).

Schoeler, Gregor. "Die Frage der schriftlichen oder mündlichen Überlieferung der Wissenschaften im frühen Islam." *Der Islam* 62 (1985): 201-230.

———, "Weiteres zur Frage der schriftlichen oder mündlichen Überlieferung der Wissenschaften im Islam." *Der Islam* 66 (1989): 38-67.

Schwarz, A.Z. *Die hebräischen Handschriften der Nationalbibliothek in Wien*. Leipzig 1925.

Sezgin, F. *Geschichte des arabischen Schriftums*. Leiden 1970-1979.

Stefani, Claudio de. "Contributi della versione araba all'edizione del testo greco del De differentiis febrium di Galeno." In: V. Boudon-Millot et al. (eds.). *Ecdotica e ricezione dei testi medici*. Naples 2006, 111-116.

Steinschneider, M. *Die arabischen Übersetzungen aus dem Griechischen*. Graz 1960.

———, *Die hebräischen Übersetzungen des Mittelalters und die Juden als Dolmetscher*. Berlin 1893; repr. Graz 1956. § 415, 9.

Strohmeier, G. "The uses of Galen in Arabic literature." In: V. Nutton (ed.). *The unknown Galen*. London, 2002, 113-120.

———, "Die christlichen Schulen in Baghdad und der alexandrinische Kanon der Galenschriften. Eine Korrektur in Ḥunains Sendschreiben an ʿAlī ibn Yaḥyā." *Oriens* 36 (2001): 268-275.

Ullmann, M. *Die Medizin im Islam*. Leiden 1970, 65-67.

Vázquez de Benito, Maria Concepcíon. *La medicina de Averroes: comentarios a*

Galeno. Salamanca, 1987.
Wallis, F. (ed.). *Medieval Medicine*. A Reader. Toronto 2010.
Walzer, R. "Codex Princetonianus Arabicus 1075," *Bulletin of the History of Medicine 28* (1954): 550-552.
Watt, John W. "The Syriac Aristotle between Alexandria and Baghdad." *Journal for Late Antique Religion & Culture 7* (2013), http://www.cf.ac.uk/share/research/centres/clarc/jlarc/contents/volume-7-2013.html
Wilkie, J.S. and Lloyd, G.E.R. "The Arabic version of Galen's De sectis ad eos qui introducuntur." *Journal of Hellenic Studies 98* (1978): 167-169.
———, "The Arabic version of Galen's Ars parva." *Journal of Hellenic Studies 101* (1981): 145.
———, "The Arabic version of Galen's De elementis secundum Hippocratem." *Journal of Hellenic Studies 102* (1982): 232-233.
Zotenberg H. (ed.) *Catalogues des Manuscrits hébreux et samaritains de la Bibliothèque Impériale*. Paris 1866.

Arabic Glossary and Index (Princeton Manuscript)

ابقراط Hippocrates 46 ← بقراط

أبيديميا ← كتاب

أثر: آثار signs 45

أذى discomfort 18 ← إحساس

ارخيجانس Archigenes 22

أسد Leo 67

أصل: أصول principles 62

أصلان two principles 62

امفيقورطن amphikurtos 63

مأمون: مأمون العاقبة sure of outcome 10,11

أنثى feminine 73

أهل family 70,71 ← خبر

آفة: آفات harmful things 2

بحث: بحث عن to investigate 13

بحث investigating 13

بحران 1,2,3,8,9,10,11,12,13,14,15,16,20,21,24
29,32,35,40,43,45,49,50,60,70,73
crisis ← علم، علامات، تكوّن، امتداد، وقت، يوم

بحرانات crises 41,45,49,50

بحراني ← أعراض، الأيّام

باحوري critical 51 ← أدوار، الأيّام

باحوري حقّ true critical 44

باحوري زور false critical 44

(بدأ) إبتدأ to begin 9,43,58,60

مبدأ onset, beginning 17,19,35,69

ابتداء beginning 40

بدر full moon 63,67

بدن body 14,27,71 ← ثقل

برج: بروج signs 23

برد chill 14

بارد ← عرق

براز excrement 10

بصر ← ظلمة

بطؤ to be slow 66

بطيء slow 56 ← حركات، أمراض

بطن ← مراق، استطلاق

بقراط Hippocrates 22,23 ← ابقراط، تقدمة

بلغم ← حمّى

بوثاغورس Pythagoras 73

بول urine 1,10

البول النضيج ripe urine 28

(بان) تبيّن 9,30,31,32,33
to be discerned, to be clear

بيّن evident, clear 2,3,11

متباين ← جزء

متباين تباينا كثيرا very distinct

تلف destruction, demise, perdition 4,26,28

تمّ to be finished 34,61

استتمّ to be complete 9

تمام completion 58

على غير تمام imperfectly 60

تامّ complete, full 10,11,75 ← دور، نَضْج

غير تامّ incomplete 29

ثقل: ثقل البدن a heaviness of the body 28

ثقل الصدغين heaviness in the temples 8

مثلّث trine

ثور Taurus 67

جالينوس Galen 16,22,25,34,35,59 ← كتاب

جدل: أصحاب الجدل dialecticians 13

جدي Capricorn 67

Hebrew Glossary and Index

אבד to die 24
אבוקראט 3,4,11,14,16,22,30
Hippocrates
אבקראט Hippocrates 9
אבר: אבר מהאברים an organ 1,4
אברים organs, limbs 8,15,16
אדמי: אדומיים red bile fevers 31
אויר ← שנוי
אות sign 12
אותות symptoms, signs 12,13,24,31
אותות הבשול 12,18
symptoms of concoction
אותות מהטבע signs from nature 13
אותות משובחים good symptoms 12
אותות רעים bad symptoms 12
אחור: איחור slowness 12
(אחר) התאחר 16,17,19,21
to come after, postpone, to come later
אמתי: אמיתי ← בחראן, גבול
אפידימיא ← ספר
ארוך prolonged 3 ← חלי
ארך to become longer 14
ארסטו/ארסטו Aristotle 31 ← חָבֵר
ארץ earth 25,29,30
באוקרסטאס Theophrastus 31
(בדל) הֶבְדֵל expulsion 8
בחראן 1,2,3,4,6,9,10,12,13,14,15,17,18,20,21,22
crisis 23,25,28 ← חֹזֶק, יום, כח, משבח
עתק, תנועה
בחראן אמיתי a true crisis 18
בחראן בטוח ורחוק מהסכנה 18
a reliable and not dangerous crisis
בחראן חסר a defective crisis 3
הבחראן הבטוח a safe crisis 18
הבחראן הוא ההתהפכות מהיר חד 1
a crisis is a fast, sudden change
הבחראן החסר the defective crisis 18
הבחראן המבואר a distinct crisis 18
הבחראן המבושר בו 18
a crisis for which warning has
been given
הבחראן המשבח a good crisis 19
הבחראן המשבח והבחראן המגונה 12
the good crisis and the bad crisis
הבחראן הרע המגונה 18
a bad, defective crisis
הבחראן השלם the complete crisis 18
והבחראן השמור 18
a trustworthy crisis
היותר משבח שבבחראן 15
the most excellent critical days
היותר רע שבבחראן 15,26
the worst of the critical
days, the worst crises
שם הבחראן נגזר מלשון היונים
והסוריאנים 1
the term “crisis” is derived
from Greek and Syriac
בחראנים crises 8
בטוח reliable, trustworthy 18,24 ← בחראן
היותר בטוח most trustworthy 19
(בטח) הובטח 7,18
to be trustworthy, to trust ← יום
בטלה: לבטלה in vain 26
ביצה ← חלמון
(בלבל) התבלבל עליו שכלו 1
to be delirious
בלגם phlegm 16
בעל: הבעל חיים המכסה חרסים 31
the sea-urchin ← ים
בריאות health 17
בשול: בישול concoction 4 ← אות, תוספת
בשול החולי 9,12
the concoction of an illness
בשורה warning 7,12,14,19,21 ← יום
(בשל) בישל to concoct 8
התבשל to be concocted 2,9
(בשר) בישר to warn, indicate 7,13,14
גאלינוס Galen 27,29 ← ספר

גב: גב הערוה ← צמיחה
גבול limit 16
גבול התכלית the limit of the climax 12
גבול יום הבחראן האמיתי 17
the limit of the real critical day
גבולים boundaries 32
שני גבולים 28,32
two boundaries, a double boundary
(גבל) הגביל to limit 13
גוף body 15,18
גלגל orb 26 ← מהלך
גלגל המזלות ecliptic 25,28,30 ←
מהלך, סב
דָּבֵק viscous 9
דבקות viscosity, overlapping 9,20,21,25
דבש ← מים
דחה to repel 18
דחות repelling, expelling 6,16,17
דחיה repelling 17
דחיית החולי repelling the disease 17
דחיית הליחות expelling the residues 8
דמוי representation 27
דפיקה palpitation 18
דפק: דפק העורקים arterial pulse 13
דק fine 9
דקות ← הנהגה
דקדק to dissolve 8
דוקדק to become fine 9
הבראה cure 2
הגלות being revealed 29
הדרגה ← יום
הויה: הוייה generation 32 ← עולם
ההויה וההפסד 16
coming to be and passing away
הוראה ← לקח
ההוראות המבשרות 14
the indications that indicate
הורג soldier 16
הזנה nutrition 10
המשכה: המשכות המניין 21
arithmetic series
הנהגה regimen, pattern 10,24 ← דקות
הנהגת החולה 10
the treatment of the patient
הנהגת המזון the regimen of food 10
ההנהגה אשר בתכלית הקצה מהדקות 11
an extremely thinning regimen
ההנהגה הדקה אשר לא תגיע בדקות
לתכליתו 11
a regimen that is thinning, but not
extremely so
ההנהגה שהיא יותר עבה 11
a more thickening regimen
מההנהגה מה שהוא בתכלית הקצה
מהדקות 10
an extremely thinning regimen
הסתערות: הסתערות חזק 15
strong agitation
הסתר: אצל הסתר הירח 29
when the moon is hidden
העמדה: העמדה וקיום being, or reality 27
העתקה motion 30
הפסד ← הויה, עולם
הפרדה separation 20
הפרדת השבועות 21
the separation between the weeks
הקדמה: הקדמת הידיעה prognosis 7,13 ←
ספר
הקף cycle 21
הקף עתותיהם their circuit 16
הקפים cycles 16,17
הקש analogy 28 ← חשבון, נקש
בהקש relative to, vis-à-vis 25,28,30
על הקש relative to 30
הרקה evacuation 1
השערה: השערת המזון 13
estimating the nutrition
התאבקות 1,2,4,9,13,15,21
struggle, agitation, combat
התהפכות change, shift 4,30 ← בחראן
התהפכות המהיר החד 4
a fast, acute change
התהפכות מהיר חד 2
a fast, sudden change
ההתהפכות הקיצי 31
the summer solstice
התוך: התוכו ההתוך שיעלם מהחוש 4
its dissolution is such that it is hidden
from the senses
התחלה beginning 21,23,28
התחלת החולי 17,19
the beginning of the illness

התחלת לקיחת הקדחת 17
the beginning of the fever
התעוררות having fits 31
זוג: זוגות pairs 17
זוגי even 23
זיעה sweat(ing) 15,18
וזה שלא תשתלח בו זיעה נגרת משתוה 19
because the sweat will not pour
forth [over his body] equally
זן to feed oneself 11
(חבר) חיבר to connect 28
התחבר to be joined 25
חָבֵר: חברי ארסטו המיוחסים אל המשאים 27
Aristotle's followers, who are linked
to the Peripatetics
חד acute 3,11 ← בחראן, התהפכות, חלי,
כליון, שנוי
חדוש 1,6,9,11,13,18
occurring, occurrence, appearing
חדות acuity 3,4 ← חלי, תכלית
חדות אל השלוח acute figuratively 3
החדות הנעתק acute from the relapse 3
חֹדֶש month 25,31 ← חשבון
חדשים months 4,5,22,24,31
חולה patient 1,7,9,10,16,28 ← הנהגה, נפל,
עזיבה
חולים patients 7
חוש ← התוך
(חזק) התחזק to be strong 17
חֹזֶק: חוזק הבחראן 4
the strength of the crisis
חָזָק strong 6,16,25 ← הסתערות, יום,
מקרה, נוע, תמונה
חיים life 1
חלוש weak 6 ← תמונה
חלי: חולי 1,4,6,9,11,12,13,17,18,28,30
illness, disease ← בשול, דחיה, התחלה,
חשבון, כלה, כליון, מין, סבה, רבות
תוספת, תכלית, תנועה
חולי ארוך long-lasting illness 4
חולי מהחוליים one of the illnesses 30
החולי החד an acute illness 4
ח(ו)ליים illnesses, diseases 3,4,6,8,18,22
← מין
החוליים הארוכים הנושנים 2
the prolonged, chronic illnesses
החוליים החדים acute illnesses 3,23,26
החוליים המיוחסים אל החדות יחס
משולח 12
the illnesses that are considered to
be acute in a general sense
החוליים הנושנים chronic illnesses 2,26
החליים הסתוים 22
the autumn or winter illnesses
חוליים הקיציים the summer illnesses 22
חלף: התחלף ימי הבחראן 18
the different critical days
חלמון: חלמון הביצה egg yolk 11
(חלק) נחלק to divide 14
חולק to be divided 25
התחלק to be divided 25
נחלק על זאת החלוקה 26
divided up in this way
חלק: חלקים parts 14
חלקה: חלוקה division 14
חלש to be weak 21
חלשה: חולשת הכח 6
the weakness of the power
חֹם/ חום fever 6,11
(חסר) התחסר waning 31
חָסֵר ← בחראן
(חפז) החפיז to trigger 16
חפזה urging 19
חפיזה haste 16
חפץ: חפץ קיא nausea 1
חצי: חצי עגלה half circuit 28 ← ירח
חקר to investigate 1
חרס: חרסים ← בעל
(חשב) נחשב 20,21,24,28
to be counted, to be computed
חשבון 21,24,25,31
calculation, computation
חשבון הקש החדש 31
a count analogous to the month
חשבון החולי 30
the computation of the illness
חשבון ימי הבחראן 14
the calculation of the critical days
חשכה: חשכת הראות dimsightedness 1
טבע nature 8,9,16,17,18,22,23,26 ← אות,
מרוצה, פעלה
טבעי ← שרש

מהירות fastness 4,12
מהירות תנועתו its swift movement 4
מהלך motion 28
מהלך הירח 15,29
the course (motion) of the moon
מהלכו בגלגלו בגלגל המזלות 29
its orb in the ecliptic orb
מוליד causing 2
מורסא inflammation 1,4,15
(מות) המית to kill
מות death 1,7
מותר residue 1,4
מזון food 10 ← הנהגה, השערה, טחינה
מזכרת casebook 22
מזל: מזלות ← גלגל
מחשבה worry, mind 16,27
מטה ← נפל
מיחד: מיוחד specific, special 23,26 ←
ענין, פעלה
מים: מי הדבש hydromel 11
מי כשך השעורים barley gruel 11
מין: מינים species 26
מין החולי the kind of disease 6
ממין החולי ר״ל מצורת החולי ומתנועתו 6
according to the kind of disease;
that is, its form and its motion
מיני החוליים the kinds of diseases 6
מלחמה battle 16
מלך: המלך הטוב a good king 19
מנה to count 25
מנוחה: המנוחה והמרגוע rest and repose 9
מנין ← המשכה
מספר number 5,26,27,28
מספרים numbers 24,26
מפרסם: מפורסם ← עליה
מציאות: מציאות שורש 27
existing as a principle
מקדם: מוקדם primary 26
מקום: מקומות הכוכבים 13
the positions of the stars
מקרה: מקרה חזק a serious accident 8
מקרים symptoms 1,18
מרגוע ← מנוחה
מרוצה: מרוצת הטבע the flow of nature 16
משאים ← חָבֵר
משבח/משובח good, best 13,16,19,21 ←
בחראן, יום, עת
יותר משובח better 9 ← אות, בחראן
משך to attract 19
משל to rule 19
משלח: משולח ← יחס
משפט verdict 1,15
משתוה equal 15 ← זיעה
משתנה changing 31
מת to die 7
מתאחר being delayed 11
מתגבר: המתגבר הרע an evil tyrant 19
מתחלף varying 30 ← שעור
נאץ to scorn
(נבט) הובט to be observed 28 ← שמר
נגוד opposition 32
נגר ← זיעה
(נהג) הנהיג עניינו to govern 19
(נוע) הניע to let (someone) exercise 9
הניע...תנועה חזקה 9
to let (someone) exercise strenuously
התנועע to move 31
נושן 3 ← חלי
(נזק) הזיק to be harmful 16,19
נח ← עזיבה
נער: נערים children 22
נעתק ← חדות
נפל: נפל החולה על המטה 17
the patient takes to his bed
נפרד odd 23
נפש: מה שאין נפש לו inanimate beings 31
(נצח) ניצח to overcome 18
(נקש) הוקש בהקש to take relative to 25
נשב to blow 29
נשג: השיג to catch up with 28,29
נשימה ← נשם
(נשם) התנשם נשימה רעה 1
to have breathing problems
(נתך) הותך 2,18,22
to dissolve, to be resolved
סב to revolve 26
העת שיסוב בו הירח בעגלתו בגלגל
המזלות 28
the time in which the moon makes
one revolution in the ecliptic
סבה cause 7,16,26
הסבה הפועלת the effective cause 16

mistake 16 פשיעה
to commit a mistake 16 פשע
פתית: פתיתי הלחם הנקי
crumbs of clean (i.e. made from
refined flour) bread
צורה ← מין
צמיחה: צמיחת השער בגב הערוה 22
reaching puberty
צף ← שתן
קדחת 3,17,26 fever ← התחלה, כח, קשי
ephemeral fever 3 קדחת יום
quartan fever 2 קדחת רביעית
quartan fever 6 הקדחת הרביעית
ardent fever 6 הקדחת השורפת
tertian fever 6 הקדחת השלישית
(הקדחת) השלישית הכפולה 17
the double quartan [fever]
fevers 3,24 קדחות
(קדם) הקדים 16,20
to come earlier, to precede
to come earlier 19 התקדם
קיא 1 emesis ← חפץ
קיום ← העמדה
summer 22,28 קיץ
קיצי ← התהפכות, חלי
shortness 3 קֹצֶר: קוצר זמן
short 3 קָצָר
short 3 קצרי הזמן
קרב: קרבים ← כאב
malignant, difficult 24,30 קשה
hardness 1,2,4,15,21 קשי: קושי
a high fever 17 קושי הקדחת
ראות ← חשכה
hidden from the eye 4 בהעלם הראות
extensiveness 16 רבוי
quadrature 32 רבוע
רבוע הירח 25,30
the quarter of the moon
quarters 25 רבועים
the quarters of the moon 25 רבועי הירח
severity of the illness 11 רבות: רבות החולי
multiples of four 26 רביעיה: רביעיות
winds 29,31 רוחות
physician 7,9,10,16 רופא
הרופא הממונה ברפואתו 16
the physician who is charged with
his cure
רחק: רחק הירח 31
the distance of the moon ← תכלית
רע 24 bad ← אות, בחראן, מתגבר
nosebleed 1 רעיפה
to treat 7 (רפא) ריפא
to be cured 7 נרפא
רפואה 9 medicine ← רופא, שתיה
to move 26 רץ
to boil 1 רתח
week 14,21,23,25 שבוע
שבועות 5,14,20,21 weeks ←
הפרדה, יום
to be good 15 (שבח) שובח
multiples of seven 26 שביעיה: שביעיות
judges 1 שופט: שופטים
שוקט ← עזיבה
שלוח ← חדות
safety 12,19 שלום
trine 32 שִׁלּוּשׁ
(שלח) השתלח ← זיעה
שלישי ← יום
to recover 24 שלם
שָׁלֵם 18,24 complete, safe ← בחראן, יום
completeness, fullness 19,31 שלמות
fullness of the moon 31 שלמות הירח
diarrhea 1,18 שלשול
שם ← בחראן
שמור 18 trustworthy ← בחראן
heaven 25,26 שמים
שמימי ← תנועה
(שמר) נשמר והובט 15
to be noticed and observed
הובט ונשמר 15
to be observed and noticed
the attendant 16 (שמש) מי שישמשהו
sun 25,28,29,30,31,32 שמש
שנה 24 year ← עת
years 4,5,22 שנים
a change in the weather 16 שנוי: שנוי האויר
השנוי המהיר החד 1
a swift, sudden change
changes 31,32 שינויים
שני ← יום
שעור: שעורים מתחלפים 26
anomalous measures

Index of Subjects

If you have any questions regarding this title, please contact:

Koninklijke Brill BV
Plantijnstraat 2
2321 JC Leiden
Email: info@brill.com

Batch number: 10703825